T0319329

Death, Modernity, and the Body

Rochester Studies in Medical History

Senior Editor: Theodore M. Brown
Professor of History and Preventive Medicine
University of Rochester

ISSN 1526-2715

Death, Modernity, and the Body

Sweden 1870–1940

EVA ÅHRÉN

TRANSLATED BY DANIEL W. OLSON

UNIVERSITY OF ROCHESTER PRESS

First published 2009
University of Rochester Press
668 Mt. Hope Avenue, Rochester, NY 14620, USA
www.urpress.com
and Boydell & Brewer Limited
PO Box 9, Woodbridge, Suffolk IP12 3DF, UK
www.boydellandbrewer.com

ISBN-13: 978-1-58046-312-6
ISBN-10: 1-58046-312-6
ISSN: 1526–2715

Library of Congress Cataloging-in-Publication Data

Åhrén, Eva.
    [Doden, kroppen och moderniteten. English]
    Death, modernity, and the body : Sweden 1870–1940 / Eva Åhrén
        p. cm. — (Rochester studies in medical history, ISSN 1526-2715 ; v. 15)
    Includes bibliographical references and index.
    ISBN-13: 978-1-58046-312-6 (hardcover : alk. paper)
    ISBN-10: 1-58046-312-6
    1. Funeral rites and ceremonies—Sweden—History. 2. Mourning customs—Sweden—History. 3. Human body—Social aspects—Sweden. 4. Human body—Symbolic aspects—Sweden. 5. Sweden—Social life and customs. I. Title.
    GT2361.A2A47   2009
    393.09485—dc22

                                                                    2009037015

A catalogue record for this title is available from the British Library.

This publication is printed on acid-free paper.
Printed in the United States of America.

For Anna-Lisa, Artur, Magnus,
and all the other friendly ghosts who haunt this book.

Contents

Illustrations

Preface

My grandmother Anna-Lisa was a remarkably wise and loving woman, and without her I would not be who I am. Even her death in 1992 changed my life by making me start thinking about death and how we deal with it. Her funeral was held in a chapel in Råcksta crematorium, a 1950s modernist brick building in a Stockholm suburb. (Typically in Sweden, after the funeral the guests leave the casket in the chapel, and the burial or scattering of the ashes takes place later.) I arrived early for the funeral to attend to practical matters and was let in through the back door, which is usually reserved for staff members. Thus, instead of entering the regular space for funeral attendees, with a lobby and a room designed for rituals and solace, I entered a workspace with tiled walls, refrigerators, conveyor belts, and incinerators. It was practical and hygienic. Men in jumpsuits were nailing flower decorations to coffin lids while a radio played pop music. A female janitor, dressed in a pink Mickey Mouse sweat suit, led me to the chapel, which she was setting up for the funeral—lighting candles and arranging flower decorations. She then left me alone and returned a little while later, dressed in black, to open the doors for the funeral guests, my family members.

The funeral was beautiful and helped me deal with my grief. But I could not stop thinking about something that sparked my curiosity about the history of death: the crematorium. It appeared to me as the perfect symbol for death in modernity: a building for dealing with practical necessities as well as funeral rites; a place with technological equipment and contemplative artworks, with noise and labor as well as stillness and prayer, with radios playing as well as organ preludes and hymns sung by mourners, with everyday routines and emotionally charged experiences.

I wanted to know when, how, and why modern, technological cremation had come into being, but I could not find the answers in books and articles. So I started researching the subject myself. First, I wrote a bachelor's thesis on the history of the Swedish cremation movement in the late nineteenth century. But that led to more questions, so I went on to graduate studies and eventually wrote a doctoral dissertation on the cultural history of death and the dead body in Sweden around the turn of the twentieth century. The dissertation was published as a book in Swedish in 2002. The present volume is a translated and revised version with a new introduction, adapted for an international audience.

Sweden's transition to modernity started considerably later than similar transitions in Britain, France, Germany, and North America. But when it hit, it was rapid and thoroughgoing, profoundly changing people's lives and deaths. Although the Swedish case is special in many respects, I hope readers of every nationality will find echoes of their own culture, history, and experience in this book, as well as inspiration to continue thinking about the never-to-be-exhausted topic of death.

Acknowledgments

I wish to thank my inspiring and supportive advisors Roger Qvarsell and Jan Garnert, my feisty fellow graduate students at Linköping University, and the superb staff and stimulating colleagues at the Royal Library in Stockholm. The research project was made possible by the financial support of the Swedish Council for Social Research (Socialvetenskapliga forskningsrådet) and the intellectual as well as emotional support of friends and family. Very special thanks to Michael Sappol, Naomi Rogers, and John Harley Warner for reading and commenting on parts of the English manuscript and for giving me valuable insights into American academic culture and history writing, and to Theodore Brown and Suzanne Guiod at the University of Rochester Press.

Chapter One

The Modernization of Death

*What could be more universal than death? Yet what an incredible vari-
ety of responses it evokes. Corpses are burned or buried, with or without
animal or human sacrifice; they are preserved by smoking, embalming, or
pickling; they are eaten—raw, cooked or rotten; they are ritually exposed
as carrion or simply abandoned; or they are dismembered and treated in
a variety of ways. . . . The diversity of cultural reaction is a measure of
the universal impact of death.*

Metcalf and Huntington, *Celebrations of Death*

The subject of this book may seem grim. Death can be an uncomfortable
topic, both emotionally and intellectually. It is a part of the human condition, difficult to deal with. An interrogation into the history of death may
evoke distress. Yet death also gives our lives meaning. We all know our lives
will end; we just don't know when, how, or why. We can ignore or acknowl-
edge this fact, but we can never escape it. Religious leaders, philosophers,
and scientists have tried to find ways of dealing with it and so have artists,
writers, composers, and filmmakers. Answers to the questions—about the
meaning of death, on how to deal with the mortality of our loved ones and
ourselves, on what will happen to us on the other side—vary from person to
person, from time to time, from culture to culture.

So what does death mean in modern Western culture? How do our conceptions of death distinguish themselves from those of our ancestors? We
die differently than our ancestors did. They tended to die young; we usually
die in old age. They tended to die from infectious diseases; we more often
die from chronic disease. They often died at home, or in places of work, or
while traveling. We most often die in hospitals, hospices, or nursing homes.
Our feelings and thoughts about death, then, necessarily differ from those of
our ancestors. For most of us, death is distant from our daily lives—death is
an abstraction. Then, when it strikes we feel confused, inadequate: our ways
of dealing with death do not always provide an adequate outlet for emotions
or satisfying rituals to perform.

In the past few decades, this uneasiness has sparked researchers in the
disciplines of history, anthropology, and ethnology, as well as sociology and
health care, to study death.[1] Much of the new scholarship has been driven

by the idea that people in the past (or other cultures) had better ways of dealing with death and has assumed that history and anthropology can provide models for reforming our death practices. Death, these scholars tell us, is "hidden" or "taboo" in modern society, in contrast to the allegedly "natural" ways people dealt with death in the past.

French historian Philippe Ariès, perhaps the best-known historian of death, claimed that death became a shameful scandal in modern society, that the dying were hidden away in hospitals and that grieving survivors were silenced to repress this scandal of death: "We ignore the existence of a scandal that we have been unable to prevent; we act as if it did not exist, and thus mercilessly force the bereaved to say nothing. A heavy silence has fallen over the subject of death."[2] Ariès, like many other writers about death, wants us to accept death, to humanize it: "Death must simply become the discreet but dignified exit of a peaceful person from a helpful society that is not torn, not even overly upset by the idea of a biological transition without significance, without pain or suffering, and ultimately without fear."[3] The study of the past is for Ariès a way of criticizing both the modern way of death and the taboo, which he sees as a result of the modern professionalization and medicalization of death and dying.

In his magisterial work *La mort et l'Occident de 1300 à nos jours,* Michel Vovelle questions Ariès's position. According to Vovelle, it is wrong to say that death is taboo when there is so much talk about it. Although the ways we deal with death have indeed changed, the subject of death has continued to be present in modernity, in its intellectual discourse and cultural representations, as well as in ritual practices. Vovelle also argues that Ariès and other modern historians of death tend to have a static view of "traditional" death practices in the past. Although some death practices are very long-lived, a cultural inertia that has much to do with long-standing demographic patterns as well as mortuary conservatism, Vovelle shows that thoroughgoing changes have occurred throughout history.[4] Historical change, then, not only means *dissolution* of traditions but also the *creation* of new practices that correspond to historically specific needs, fears, and conceptions of death, in modernity as well as in former times.

In this book, I intend to show that during the late nineteenth and early twentieth centuries, a period of intense sociocultural transformation, Swedish death practices and ways of handling human remains changed considerably. Yet I have found nothing to indicate that this led to a decreased respect, an increased fear of death, or a taboo.[5] I will not try to evaluate historical changes in terms of gains and losses; my purpose is to describe and contextualize the changing ways of dealing with the bodies of the dead. Also, I have not tried to be comprehensive—instead, I have chosen a limited number of aspects to study, and there are many more that could be explored.

The modernization of death went hand in hand with the modernization of society and culture at large. It was driven by a desire to be modern (secular, efficient, scientific, hygienic, rational), to change traditional death customs in accordance with modern ideals. Surviving family members became death service consumers, contributing to this modernization of death together with undertakers, burial reformers, health reformers, state administrators, church officials, and scientists.

The dead body is charged with different, sometimes opposing meanings in different historical and cultural contexts. The various actors who concern themselves with the dead body ascribe it meaning within a wide framework. Thus from the viewpoint of social planning, a body can be a sort of refuse that must be disposed of (a pollutant or contaminant). At the same time, for those in grief it is the emotionally charged remains of a relative or a friend, and for the funeral director it represents a source of income. For the pathologist and the archaeologist, the dead body, or parts of it, is an object of study. These are only a few of the conceivable meanings that may be given to the dead body.

Over time these meanings change. They are renegotiated within the framework of historical givens and take on different forms, depending upon factors such as the age, gender, class, ethnic background of the deceased and the observer. Within a single culture, the ways of handling dead criminals, suicide victims, and enemies differ from those used for children or people in power.[6]

What, then, does the opening quotation have to do with this topic? It seems to deal only with exotic and foreign cultures, and some of the methods of dealing with dead bodies it describes are undeniably foreign to Western culture. Yet others are not: the bodies of the dead are burned or buried in the earth; they are preserved by embalming; they are weighed, measured, and their entrails are examined; they are divided into smaller portions and pickled; they are put into special boxes, decorated and displayed to the public. Some ways of dealing with the dead have ancient origins, while others are fairly recent. While the impact of death is universal, the cultural manifestations of death are always culturally and historically situated.

The Meaning of Death

An array of rules governs the handling of the dead in modern societies. While some of these rules arise out of practical or bureaucratic considerations, most are ritual or symbolic. Even seemingly rational rules for the handling of corpses may have symbolic, magical, and ritual components. For anthropologists, the study of death rituals is a central subject, a way to understand cultures and worldviews, and it has been so throughout the history of the discipline.[7]

Why do dead human bodies have to be handled in compliance with culturally specific rules? According to the classic explanation by Arnold van Gennep in 1909, people link certain major events with a series of ritual acts, which he named rites of passage (*rites de passage*).[8] These events—birth, sexual maturity, marriage, and death—are occasions when a person's social standing changes, often tied to bodily changes. Such rites mark and reshape the relationship between individual and society. Following a systematic comparison of such rituals, Gennep argued that rites of passage are often organized according to a pattern. The person or persons at the center of the rite first undergoes a *separation* from the surrounding society. Next, the *transition* or passage itself occurs, and a symbolic border is crossed. Finally, the person or persons who have undergone the rite are *incorporated* into society in their new standing or position. Rites of passage are often arranged as a trip or journey, during which one passes through a concrete symbol of transition, such as a threshold or doorway.

Although every funeral is in some ways unique, one can describe the typical course of a funeral in rural Sweden around 1900, based on descriptions in the archive of the Nordic Museum in Stockholm, in accordance with van Gennep's theories. The deceased was *separated* from the living through a series of rites involving the taking of farewells, washing, enshrouding, placement in a casket, and often placement in a separate and specially decorated room. The *transition* occurred in the form of a journey from the home of the deceased, where participants in the rite gathered to follow the deceased to the cemetery. Since the usual time for burial was before the Sunday church service, and more than one burial could occur on the same day, the different funeral parties waited for one another and then carried their caskets through the cemetery gateway in a certain order, based on the class, gender, and age of the deceased. Through the funeral, the deceased was *given a new position:* the series of rites was completed when the deceased was given the status of dead.[9]

During the time between the moment of death and burial, the dead body has an uncertain status. The deceased exist on a border between the world of the living, to which they recently belonged, and the world of the dead, to which they do not yet belong. This borderline existence, this "liminal" nature, makes the body dangerous for the living.[10] Death disturbs the social order by tearing an individual from his or her context. The function of the rites of death and burial is thus to reestablish order and create meaning out of death.[11] The corpse embodies the disorder created by death and is thus conceived to be dangerous. Dead bodies are ascribed powers: they bring health and sickness, fortune and misfortune.[12]

The belief that contact with dead bodies can bring contagion or contamination goes far beyond our own culture and history, as anthropologist

Mary Douglas has shown.[13] The concept of pollution is not absolute. What is understood to be dirty is dependent upon ideas of order. Concepts of contagion, according to Douglas, are analogies or symbols for social relations. Contagion is associated with anomalies and things that have unclear status in a culture. Filth, contagion, and uncleanliness point to order and disorder, being and lack of being, form and formlessness, life and death.[14]

According to Douglas, dead bodies have an anomalous or borderline status. Borders are always dangerous, especially when they relate to bodily stages, but the place of danger varies from culture to culture. Each has its own special risks and problems. Which bodily borderline states, excretions, or openings are associated with filth, contagion, danger, and power depends upon the relationships the body reflects in a specific culture. The dangerous is charged with meaning.[15] Attitudes toward dead (or living) bodies can thus provide clues to the fundamental concepts of a culture. Changing attitudes are linked to changing concepts. People's ways of dealing with the remains of the dead are charged with meaning. If the ways of handling dead bodies change, so do the conceptions and beliefs of those who perform these acts.

My approach to this subject is cross-disciplinary: historical and anthropological. My sources are varied: newspapers, textbooks, popular science, technical drawings, photographs, and more.[16] I want to "anthropologize" history.[17] In this effort, Clifford Geertz's concept of culture has proved especially useful.[18]

In "Thick Description: Toward an Interpretive Theory of Culture," Geertz defined culture as actions that create meaning. This occurs communicatively, through speech, text, artifacts, and actions. The meanings thus created are open and social and available for interpretation. The anthropologist describes and interprets signs or symbols: culture is a context in which symbols can be described so they can be understood.[19] To study the *inner system* of these symbols is too abstract; the symbols receive their meaning in a social context. Culture is thus not a metaphysical phenomenon but a social one.[20]

Geertz warned that it is important to avoid becoming bogged down in, on one hand, too subjective interpretation and, on the other, overly rigid systematizations.[21] One should maintain a close relationship to the subject matter, neither rising too far above it nor digging too deeply below it. The goal of an interpretive researcher is not to answer the deepest questions of human existence but rather *to make other people's answers to these questions accessible.*[22]

My approach, however, is not primarily anthropological but historical. According to Paul Ricoeur, the work of the historian is to forge narrative reconstructions.[23] Both fiction and history have this possibility: the capacity to reveal and transform narratives of actual actions and suffering.[24] Knowledge about history is gained through *traces*. The trace is a left-behind remainder that represents the past and which the historian interprets. It has a special double status in that it exists as a marker in the present while its historical context has disappeared. However, only to the extent that it is regarded as evidence of something absent does it gain the character of being a trace. In the historical discourse, the trace has the function of existing "in place of" the past, which is absent from the historian's present. References to the reality of the past are thus indirect; they pertain to knowledge gained through the interpretation of traces.[25] Traces of the past are *the only evidence* the historian has in the search for knowledge about the past. The historian's knowledge is always characterized by *the indirect* and cannot be separated from its nature of reconstruction.[26]

The idea that culture is not subordinate to the social or material is vital. Within historical scholarship, there has been a shift from the sociological toward the cultural. As Ricoeur tells us, this shift does not necessarily mean the historian has lost ties to the actions and suffering of human reality. On the contrary, it is important not to exchange the reductionist view of social history (that culture only reflects social reality) for an idealistic cultural view, which ignores material acts and productions. Both Geertz and Ricoeur point to the need for empirical research to keep hold of reality.

Geertz maintains that culture is open. Although it is intangible, it exists, not least of all in people's minds. Its expressions exist in this world, and these expressions are our objects of study. Our task is not to seek their ontological status but rather their meaning, that is, what is said through their occurrence.[27] If we take Geertz and Ricoeur seriously, the goal of (historical) interpretation is not to depict the reality *behind* the traces. Rather, the meaning lies *in* the traces themselves. The goal is to reach an understanding through interpretation, *to see something as something.*[28] This is in fact the historian's only possibility. The object of study is not and cannot be the historical reality, since it no longer exists. Instead, the historian's objects are remainders, traces, of actions in history. The work is interpretive and the knowledge is indirect. The historian does not reproduce reality but rather constructs it through meaning-creating work.

The Modernization of Sweden

Beginning with Karl Marx, Emile Durkheim, and Max Weber, writers in the humanities and social sciences have analyzed, discussed, and criticized what it means to be modern, what modernity is about, what constitutes modern societies. I am not going to apply any grand theory of modernity here. Neither will I take sides in the debate on whether modernity is essentially a good, emancipatory force of change or a destructive, alienating one. Instead I will apply a very pragmatic, historical perspective: I take modernity to mean both a time period and its primary characteristics. Modernity is the historical era marked by industrialization, urbanization, secularization, globalization, and capitalism. It is characterized by a high valuation of concepts such as progress, rationalism, scientific objectivity, innovation, individualism, and freedom from the controlling aspects of tradition.[29]

Modernization is the process by which modern society comes into being, a historically tangible process of change. But it can also mean the process by which a certain phenomenon is changed to fit modern values and practices, such as "the modernization of death." In this book, my focus is on the 1870s through the 1930s, a period of Swedish history marked by the intensification of modernization and great changes at all levels of society. The transformation of Swedish death practices, then, is a small part of a larger historical process: the formation of modern society.

Industrialization took off considerably later in Sweden than in England, France, and Germany. It was not until the end of the nineteenth century that Sweden began in earnest the transformation from an agriculturally based state to a modern industrial nation. The population began to move from the countryside to the cities, and a new industrial working class developed. As late as the interwar period, however, the majority of Sweden's population still made its living from agriculture. Slowly but steadily, modernization changed the conditions of people's lives, not least through structural and communications breakthroughs such as railroads, steamboats, electricity, and, eventually, telephones, radio, and cars.[30] Innovations such as organized garbage collection, running water, and the gradual replacement of privies by flush toilets also changed people's everyday lives, perhaps especially for women. Relations between social classes and individuals were influenced by the new life patterns, as were relations between the sexes. Several phases of democratization took place, but the process was spiked with conflict, strikes, and class struggle.

This reconfiguration of people's lives did not follow a direct course or obvious line of development toward the better, as the proponents of modernization imagined it would.[31] The history of modernization is not only about how economics, technology, and politics transformed society and people's lives. The transformation was driven in a tangible way by people whose ideas, vision, and intellectual reasoning influenced the course of history. For instance, the 1930s concept of Sweden as a "people's home" providing benefits for all citizens grew from multifaceted ideas that centered on the contradictory pairs of city/country and individual/collective. Acceptance of the city and individuality was related to ideals of efficiency, order, and hygiene. Yet Swedish modernity also incorporated seemingly antimodern ideals such as community, solidarity, and closeness to nature.[32]

Health and hygiene played an important role in modernization discourse. These values were manifested in an increased commitment to medical research, the building of institutions for health care, mass circulation of advice on health, forced sterilizations, and more.[33] In the late nineteenth century an intense campaign occurred for hygiene in Sweden. The idea of cleanliness was applied to new areas, reaching far beyond the surface of the individual body to the body of society itself. This process reached ever deeper into the human body and in part took the form of racial hygiene, or eugenics.[34] But even as late as the 1930s, although the modernization of Sweden was rapid, the lack of hygiene among certain populations could still be conceived as a problem. Ludvig "Lubbe" Nordström, today best known for his 1938 radio reportage series *Lort-Sverige* (*Filth-Sweden*), praised modernization and condemned filth, degeneration, and the traditional rural way of life. He praised medical doctors who struggled to achieve public health, and he dreamed of a sort of "normalized showcase society, symmetrical and standardized." Nordström's ideals agreed in large part with the values of the Swedish middle class, even if he sometimes expressed them more pointedly.[35]

The Church of Sweden, a Protestant Lutheran state church, dominated Swedish religious life, although some evangelical revival movements gained large followings during the nineteenth century. From 1860, Swedish citizens could choose to join any other church (but until 1951 they were not allowed to leave the Church of Sweden without becoming a member of another church). Parish churches, and their Sunday morning Mass, were hubs of social and cultural life in rural Sweden, but their influence slowly diminished with urbanization. The secularization of modern social life progressed hand in hand with the increasingly strong cultural and institutional position of science. A scientifically based worldview largely replaced a generally accepted Lutheran orthodoxy or was integrated with more modern and open forms of Christian faith.[36]

In this book I discuss a number of themes, or aspects, of modernity, sometimes explicitly, sometimes as subtexts. The first is that of the tension between traditional and modern life and worldviews. The second is that of the results of urbanization and the contrasts between city and countryside. The third is how variables of gender, class, and ethnicity set the frameworks for people's patterns of action and thought. The fourth centers on increased efficiency, specialization, professionalization, and institutionalization as expressions of modernity.

Cultural Practices of Death in Sweden

The true classic on customs and practices surrounding death and burial in Sweden is *När döden gästar: Svenska folkseder och svensk folktro i samband med död och begravning* (*When Death Comes to Visit: Swedish Folk Customs and Beliefs Connected with Death and Burial*), published in 1937. The author, Louise Hagberg, was a folklore researcher who had worked at the Nordic Museum since 1891, first as a secretary and later as a researcher.[37] *När döden gästar* is a remarkable work of seven hundred pages, in which Hagberg reports on hundreds of customs throughout Sweden based on archived records of conversations with older "bearers of tradition," the published works of other folklore researchers, and Hagberg's own research trips within Sweden. *När döden gästar* is a unique study of "traditional" death customs.[38]

Hagberg worked from a set of theoretical and methodological suppositions that are no longer in vogue.[39] In Hagberg's day, the collection of surviving folk beliefs and customs was considered urgent, since rapid modernization was eradicating original and genuine aspects of Swedish culture. Hagberg sought to reconstruct the most ancient portions of Swedish folk belief. She felt she could do so by studying contemporary customs and practices and comparing them to archaeological finds and observations of "primitive" cultures. Researchers believed the old ideas and rituals survived in new forms and as cultural "relics," which with time had become increasingly meaningless. They thought the study of surviving cultural practices and artifacts would uncover traces that linked them to more ancient forms. The more widespread a custom was (in Scandinavia, Europe, or throughout the entire world), the more original it was believed to be: "In the customs of death, the most seminal aspects of all the old beliefs and traditions have been preserved. We find the original religious ideas collected in these beliefs."[40] As a result, Hagberg gives the impression that folk culture was static and undifferentiated, timeless.

När döden gästar thus can serve both as secondary literature and as source material. It depicts "traditional" customs and practices surrounding death and burial. But it also testifies to the currency of ideas about death in Sweden during the first half of the twentieth century (those held by Hagberg and her contemporaries), as well as the relationship of ethnology to "the people" and their traditions. Here, it will be used to provide an overview of death practices in premodern Sweden and as a window to the suppositions and principles of collection that guided the organization of the archives in early-twentieth-century Sweden.[41]

According to Hagberg, the subject of death had to be treated with special care. In old Swedish folk belief it was dangerous to talk about death. Death was too serious a subject to be mentioned in daily conversation. To speak of it moved speaker and listener into a special realm. Because of the "reluctance about this subject, when it enters into conversation," Hagberg suggested, it had been inaccessible to folklorists.[42] Both researchers and informants met with this reluctance about the subject, she further argued. If so, then perhaps death did not become a taboo subject during the twentieth century as part of the process of modernization. To me, the modern "denial of death" seems to be a new form of an old phenomenon.

The most complete recent cultural history of death in Sweden is found in the works of Nils-Arvid Bringéus.[43] His writings abound with insights, but

Bringéus tends to be overly judgmental of modern deathways. Like many other researchers who have written about death, Bringéus is driven by the idea that contemporary ways of dealing with the deceased are faulty and need to be changed and that we can learn from the past.

In *Livets högtider* (*Ceremonies of Life*), Bringéus wrote about the celebrations and rites in Swedish cultural history that mark transitions in human lives, from christenings to funerals.[44] He shows that customs and practices have changed over the course of history and that these changes are linked to larger cultural and social changes, without reducing them to simple reflections of economic, political, or other conditions.

Customs and practices create meaning out of the bodily phases of transition of human life. Bringéus argued that cultural manifestations have gradually become distanced in time and space from the physical event of death they ritualize.[45] For example, in contemporary Sweden, funerals often take place several weeks after the death; interment of the ashes may take place up to a year after cremation. The custom of holding watch over the newly deceased began to disappear during the eighteenth century, and in Sweden today, open casket funerals are rare.[46]

Ceremonies marking the phases of life are sensual experiences, and this is no less true of funerals, with their bouquets, ringing of church bells, organ music, and coffee and other refreshments. Funerals are occasions when emotion is expressed and externalized. We associate them primarily with crying, grieving, and sympathy; but since funeral celebrations in earlier periods could last several days, we can imagine that the mood had time to shift. The wake or funeral party was a place where relatives and friends met and reaffirmed their connections. These sensual aspects have changed radically. The organization of funerals, and other ceremonies of the phases of life, depends greatly on those who plan them, or, in the words of Bringéus, "the directors and producers of life's ceremonies."[47] In the early 1900s, undertakers began to offer an increasing number of services as part of their business; thus the modern funeral began taking shape.

Life-phase ceremonies are also used to enforce authority and exercise power. In Sweden, all deaths have been registered since the mid-eighteenth century. Since then, an ever-increasing number of regulations and protocols have come into being. The death of a human being can serve as an ideological breaking point, an occasion for the ceremonial expression of worldviews and ideas. At the same time, death can function as a marker of social boundaries, delineating age, gender, and class as well as regional, linguistic, religious, and national identity. The custom of church bell ringing in southern Sweden is one example. The ringing of bells finely marked the social identity of the deceased (when to ring the bells, how many times, and other considerations). A similar cultural logic governed mourning clothes.[48]

Medicine and the Dead Body

The knowledge that can be gained from studying dead bodies, cutting them open to scrutinize them in ever-greater detail, finding out what killed the person, or trying out surgical procedures has been of great importance to Western medicine.[49] This became increasingly so in the nineteenth century, when the number of dead bodies used by the medical professions rose steadily—in part because of an increase in the number of medical students, in part for scientific reasons. As Michel Foucault has shown in *The Birth of the Clinic: An Archaeology of Medical Perception,* the ways of practicing pathological anatomy in Paris in the beginning of the nineteenth century brought a new set of attitudes to Western medicine. Disease came to be analyzed "from the point of view of death," by systematically opening up corpses and comparing the results to diagnoses made during the person's lifetime (what is known as the anatomo-clinical method). "From the point of view of death, disease has a land, a mappable territory, a subterranean, but secure place, where its kinships and its consequences are formed; local values define its forms. Paradoxically, the presence of the corpse enables us to perceive it living . . ."[50] As pathological anatomy grew, so did the number of corpses used for dissections in teaching, research, and forensic investigation. Chapter 2 discusses the use of dead bodies in medicine in Sweden and how the attitudes of anatomists and pathologists differed from those of the laity.

The rising demand for corpses to dissect in medical schools and the increased frequency of pathological and forensic autopsies aroused public concern. In the eighteenth century the only corpses sent to Swedish anatomical institutions were those of executed criminals, suicides, and illegitimate children. In the nineteenth century other groups were added: people who died in prisons, workhouses, poorhouses, hospitals, and asylums. Patients who died in care institutions were required to undergo postmortem examination. A hierarchy of importance was established: forensic autopsies were given highest priority, followed by clinical autopsies and anatomical dissections.

The public generally opposed the opening up of dead bodies. The government therefore was beset by the conflicting demands of doctors and the public. Some traces of these conflicts over the right to use corpses appear in medical records but not in legal records, unlike nineteenth-century Britain and America.[51] There is no evidence of body snatchers, murders to obtain corpses, or riots against medical schools in Sweden. The public disapproved of dissection because it was seen as a kind of postmortem punishment. People also disapproved of the idea that a dead human body could be made useful. Dissection transforms the deceased person into a medical object, something to be looked at as a curiosity or cut open as though it were a piece of meat, which violated funerary honor and ritual practice. This opposition notwithstanding, little by little medical postmortem examinations became accepted as a routine part of the practices associated with death—a modern rite of passage.

Displaying the Dead Body

Preparing specimens to be used in research and education was a central practice in anatomical and pathological institutions in the nineteenth and early twentieth centuries, in Sweden as elsewhere in the Western world. Visualization of bodily structures played a crucial role in the production of anatomical knowledge. Work in various forms of visual media (such as drawings, photographs, charts, tables, models in wax or plaster, wet or dried specimens) constituted an important part of a medical scientist's professional repertoire.

At the same time specimens preserved or represented through various techniques were on display in professional anatomical and pathological museums, the general public could see similar objects on display at the popular anatomy shows and wax museums. These exhibitions often displayed dissected bodies or body parts and disease conditions modeled in the extremely realistic substance of wax. At times, (parts of) real dead bodies were on display, such as Egyptian child mummies, malformed fetuses in formalin, a drinker's stomach, or the dried skin of an African "native." Death was also on display in the form of death masks of well-known personalities, tableaux of murders and executions, and celebrities on their deathbeds. The freak show was a related form of popular culture, which also profited from objectifying odd or monstrous bodies. Wax museums, freak shows, and medical collections of specimens share a common history, dating back to old collections of curiosities.

During the nineteenth century, deformed bodies came to be defined less as marvels or freaks of nature and more as pathological deviations. Medical discourse dissociated itself from the commercial spectacles of the human body and transformed freakery into pathology. Freak shows and wax museums that were parts of the visual culture at the turn of the twentieth century all but disappeared in the interwar period. In Sweden professional medical museums disappeared around the same time. The heyday of the medical museum—the decades around 1900—coincided with that of wax museums, freak shows, and popular anatomy exhibitions.

Chapter 3 shows that medical representations and commercial displays of (dead) bodies are connected through a series of representing and ordering practices. They are part of the same visual culture, centered on death, deviance, and the body.

Undertakers Take Over

Chapter 4 deals with ways of preparing the dead body for the funeral and how these practices changed with Sweden's modernization. Ritualized customs, such as washing and clothing the deceased, used to be the work of local women, especially in rural cultures. The manner of preparing corpses was motivated by both practical considerations and magical beliefs. For example, it was believed that nail and hair clippings should be destroyed and that the water used to wash the dead had to be dealt with in elaborate ways to prevent the dead from haunting the realm of the living. The practice of washing the dead body was often motivated by the idea that the deceased should be clean and proper when presented to the Lord. It was a symbolic cleansing, separating the dead from the living and preparing the deceased for incorporation into the community of the dead. At the same time, the custom had aesthetic, theatrical aspects; it prepared the body for the leave-taking rituals.

In the late nineteenth century there were very few undertakers in Sweden, even in Stockholm.[52] The custom of engaging professionals to take care of the dead body gained ground among the well-to-do in cities and towns and then gradually spread to rural areas. Undertakers often started off as coffin makers, progressively extending their business to include more commodities and services. The growth of undertaking businesses accelerated in the interwar period, and by the middle of the twentieth century this modern institution was well established.

The growth of undertaking is often characterized as a professionalization of death, which implies that undertakers' services differ essentially from traditional ritual practices. I will argue that the practices of undertakers also serve important ritual functions. Customs were modified and changed with modernization, but the fact that professional practitioners performed some of them did not diminish their ritual value.

Memorial Photography

Postmortem photography—that is, photographic portraits of dead persons—arose in the 1850s and 1860s, at the same time as portrait photography. It evolved from the older practice of deathbed portraiture, which, through photography, became affordable for ordinary people.[53]

Chapter 5 deals with Swedish postmortem photography. Postmortem photos serve the purpose of memorializing the deceased but also convey other meanings. The photos fall into two genres. The first records the funeral as a social event: families and funeral guests are gathered around the coffin. These pictures are most often taken outdoors in a rural setting. The second is more singularly focused on the deceased and serves as memorial portraiture. Photos of this kind were taken in bourgeois parlors as well as in peasants' cottages. In Sweden the vast majority of postmortem photographs depict the deceased in a coffin.

Despite the modernity of the photographic technique and the long tradition of deathbed portraiture, this type of image did not survive in the visual culture of the twentieth century. Death disappeared from family albums, a fact related to the decline in the customs of viewing the dead and of keeping the dead at home until the day of the funeral. But it also reveals a new, specifically modern sensitivity or aversion to looking at this kind of picture of the dead. The dead we meet in the visual culture of late modernity are either fictional, as in crime or horror movies, or anonymous, as in news reports from scenes of war or terror.

Cremation and Modernity

In the late nineteenth century, members of the Swedish liberal bourgeois elite advocated cremation. The members of the Swedish Cremation Society—which started activities in 1882—were mainly male physicians, industrialists, engineers, and architects, as well as artists and intellectuals. Arguments for the new form of disposal of dead bodies were often based on hygiene, an important concept and driving force for the modernization process at large. Chapter 6 deals with the introduction and establishment of cremation in Sweden.

There is a special problem concerning dead human bodies: on the one hand, the corpse is refuse matter, and on the other, it is supposed to be handled with reverence and respect. The dead body is a dangerous source of pollution, but at the same time it is the remains of a human being, transformed by death into something with different qualities, associated with holiness and mystery. This duality of the dead body had a major influence on cremationists' sometimes ardent commitment. Refusing to accept the horrifying decomposition of the corpse, they wanted to take command, if not of death itself, at least of its consequences. The activities of the cremation societies also reflect the different meanings a dead body had. Their objectives were to develop the practicalities of cremation (e.g., technology, hygienic and forensic regulations), as well as to create suitable rituals and symbols.

During the nineteenth century the sense of disgust over decomposing corpses intensified. Cremation was an instrument for controlling the destructive forces of nature. By means of steel, fire, and engineering, the horrors of putrefaction were overpowered. In the vision of cremationists, purity, enlightenment, and activity defeated disintegration, darkness, and passivity.

Attitudes toward death and the dead body underwent profound changes during the period of Sweden's intense modernization around the turn of the twentieth century (as did many other aspects of culture and society). This book's empirical chapters (chapters 2–6) deal with the changes in death practices. I will argue that ways of handling dead bodies changed to meet the specific fears and conceptions of death in modernity and that the variability of attitudes toward death corresponded to culturally constituted, historically changing needs.

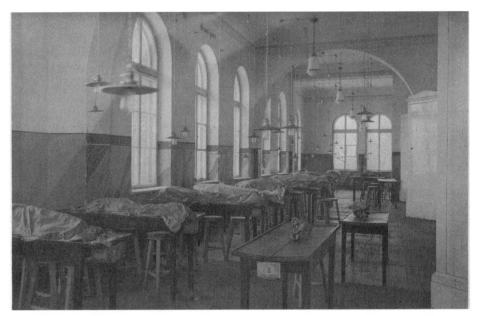

Figure 1. A dissection room with neat rows of cadavers waiting to be uncovered by medical students; Riga, Latvia, 1925 (photographer unknown). From a photo album that belonged to Gaston Backman, Swedish professor of anatomy. Maps and Prints, Uppsala University Library.

Chapter Two

On the Usefulness of the Dead

With a fine-edged iron knife almost like a common table knife, the brain is now divided into a number of centimeter-thick slices, in the same way that a loaf of bread is cut into slices.

Salomon Eberhard Henschen, "Om den tekniska
undersökningen af hjärnan: Några anmärkningar"

The dissection room at the Department of Anatomy at Lund University was built in 1897. An inscription above the entrance reads HIC LOCUS EST UBI MORS GAUDET SUCCURRERE VITAE, meaning "This is the place where death is pleased to assist life."[1] Anatomists often regarded their work in this way; dead bodies were construed as useful because they could be examined scientifically. Science made death into a servant of life. This attitude is probably as old as the study of anatomy itself, and it was frequently expressed in the late 1800s.

Statements about death as a servant of science and life are found primarily in formal speeches and inscriptions. But just how did death serve science, and why did science in the nineteenth century take death into its service to an extent never before imagined?

The attitudes of scientists toward the dead body differed markedly from those of the general public. While the dead body was deemed useful in the service of medicine, there was widespread public disapproval of all forms of cutting into dead bodies, which was regarded as a desecration. This chapter examines what these different attitudes represented and the extent to which they were reflected in legislation, and it concludes with a discussion of power over the body in relation to modernity.

Anatomical Dissections

The word "dissection" is derived from the Latin word for "to cut," *secare*, in combination with the prefix *dis-*, which means "apart." The word "anatomy" also means to cut apart, but it comes from the Greek.[2] This is exactly what is meant here: to cut up dead bodies in order to study their structure.[3]

As discussed in chapter 1, the use of dead bodies was of central importance to the development of medical science during the nineteenth century. Although anatomical instruction had long been a part of medical education, it became even more important as a result of more widespread application of pathology and the anatomo-clinical method.[4] At the same time that the number of medical students rose, hands-on dissection practice was introduced to the curriculum. The need for bodies for research and education increased, as did the need for an infrastructure for handling bodies and body parts. At the beginning of the nineteenth century, Sweden had two medical faculties for the education of physicians, located at the old universities in Uppsala and Lund. In addition, the Collegium Medicum in Stockholm had established an educational program for surgeons and field doctors, which later developed into the Karolinska Institute. The Karolinska Medico-Chirurgiska Institutet (the Karolinska Medico-Surgical Institute), as it was first called, was founded in 1810. While the ideals of natural philosophy still dominated the older medical faculties, the Karolinska Institute cultivated the new concept of scientific medicine. Disagreements arose, especially between Uppsala's leading man, Israel Hwasser, and the Karolinska's internationally renowned leader, chemist Jöns Jacob Berzelius.[5]

At the Karolinska Institute, anatomy was highly valued, and efforts were made to develop the institute's anatomical instruction. This resulted in part from the scientific attitude toward medicine and in part from the fact that the institute primarily educated surgeons. (The education of surgeons was more practical and hands-on than that of physicians. In an era without effective painkillers and anesthesia, surgeons needed a thorough knowledge of anatomy and extensive practice cutting into bodies, which would allow them to complete operations quickly.) Corpses were also more accessible in Stockholm than in the rest of Sweden because of its greater population and its many hospitals, workhouses, prisons, and similar institutions.[6] In any case, anatomical instruction at the Karolinska Institute became a magnet for medical students from Uppsala and Lund, who demanded better anatomical instruction than their schools could offer. Earlier, many had studied abroad to gain more practical skills in anatomy than were offered at the two universities. Because the Karolinska Institute was not granted the right to graduate medical students until 1873, however, these students had to return to their home universities to complete their degrees.[7]

In his memoirs, Magnus Huss, professor of medicine at the Karolinska Institute during the period 1840–60 and chief surgeon at Stockholm's Serafimer Hospital, related that in 1829 he and eleven other medical students at Uppsala were forced to undertake dissections without the guidance of an instructor:

From Stockholm, one—I repeat, *one*—corpse was procured. We were to begin with myology (the study of muscles). The study thereof proceeded thusly, that *one* of us—the later so eminent surgeon Swalin—undertook the dissection, while we other eleven stood around him and observed. Sometimes he had dissected the section he was working on before our arrival. Another student would read from Hempel's description of the section of the body at hand; and finally, the same was reviewed on prints which hung on the wall. Thus only one of the twelve students had actually laid a hand upon our chief object, namely, the anatomical dissection work itself. The result of this fact was that most of us left Uppsala in order to study anatomy under Anders Retzius [at the Karolinska Institute] in Stockholm.[8]

It was also difficult to obtain clinical experience in places other than Stockholm. The capital city had more hospitals and other care-giving institutions where students from the Karolinska Institute could gain clinical experience and where the anatomo-clinical method was practiced.[9] Under Huss's leadership, the first program of clinical instruction was established, according to what he called the anatomical-pathological method. Huss described the three stages of clinical instruction: first, the diagnosis is made, based on "physical methods of examination," that is, auscultation and percussion; second, a suitable treatment is given; and finally, if the patient died, "an examination of the information provided by opening the body, as well as comparisons between [this information] and the symptoms which had occurred during the patient's life."[10] Serafimer Hospital and the Karolinska Institute were the first institutions in Sweden to use this method of instruction, and they held to it firmly and further developed it. Great importance was placed on students gaining personal, hands-on experience through dissection.

During the seventeenth century, the usual procedure for a dissection was that a so-called prosector was responsible for opening the dead body and pointing out its organs while a professor lectured on the results. The dissection of a body in the presence of an audience could continue for several consecutive days. In Bologna, Italy, public dissections were held during Carnival and were attended by masked Carnival merrymakers during a ten-day period.[11] Public dissections in Sweden were less theatrical, although they drew an audience beyond the medical students and journeyman field surgeons enrolled in the course.[12]

By the time of Magnus Huss's anatomy classes, public dissections had long been done away with, but even in the 1820s many doctors never laid their hands on a dead human body during their education. By the end of the nineteenth century, though, the situation was entirely different, and the Karolinska Institute's approach to instructional dissections had more or less won out. In 1884, Edvard Clason, a professor of anatomy at Uppsala University, formulated an answer to the question "How should one dissect?": "So that one thereby procures upon the basis of personal observations the most complete knowledge possible of the human body."[13]

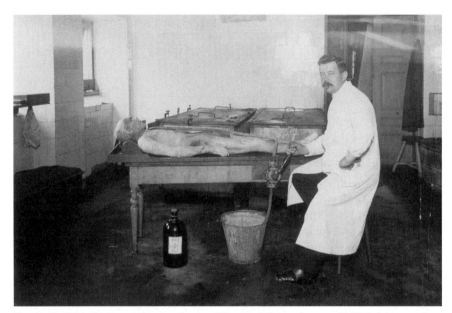

Figure 2. Embalming at the Academy of Surgery, Copenhagen, 1910 (photographer unknown). Medical Museion, University of Copenhagen.

Under the direction of their prosector and professor, medical students carried out dissections in large halls equipped with rows of dissection tables. According to Israel Holmgren, who taught anatomy under Clason at Uppsala in the early 1890s, four students would often share one corpse. First, the muscles were uncovered; next came the blood vessels, which were clearly marked by having been injected with red lead; then were the nerves; and finally, the contents of the torso were revealed.[14]

Dissections were carried out in different ways, depending upon the goals of the instruction. For a class in topographical anatomy, the most important factor was the position of organs relative to one another, and the procedure had to be carried out differently than, for example, a class in musculature and ligaments. Rarely was an entire body used; rather, a certain portion of a body or an organ was chosen for the class. These portions were prepared by the prosector or by one of the custodians who managed the handling of corpses in the department, embalmed them, transported them to and from mortuaries and cellars, took care of remains left after the dissection, sharpened the instruments, and so on. In a photograph from Copenhagen about 1910, a custodian is shown in the process of embalming. The man sits laconically next to a dead body, smoking, with a bucket and a bottle of chemicals next to him. In the background are large tubs, used to preserve bodies (see figure 2).[15]

Legislation and Anatomists' Need for Corpses

Anatomists and pathologists in the nineteenth and early twentieth centuries seem to have had no doubts that their work was of benefit to society and necessary for scientific progress. The general public's reluctance or fear regarding tampering with death was dismissed as superstition and ridiculed, opposed, or simply ignored. Discussion or reflection about the ethical dimensions of the work and conflicts with the general public may have occurred among medical scientists, but they were not recorded in textbooks, scientific articles, or case studies. I have interpreted doctors' attitudes by reading between the lines and studying tangible actions.

Legislation regarding the handling of dead bodies changed over time, and the laws reveal much about contemporary attitudes toward dead bodies. The need for corpses for dissection purposes grew successively during the nineteenth century as a result of the increasingly strong position of science within education and research. Swedish legislators made efforts to balance the demands of anatomists against a skeptical public opinion. The formulations of the laws thus reveal conflicts as well as attitudes and actions prevailing at the time of their enactment. To understand how and on what grounds anatomists' access to corpses was regulated, a short historical overview is necessary.[16]

During the seventeenth century, only executed criminals were turned over to anatomists. Eventually, the number of corpses available to anatomists became insufficient because of increased demand, and during the eighteenth century other opportunities arose. A royal letter from 1747 established that in addition to the bodies of executed criminals, the universities in Uppsala, Lund, and Turku and the Collegium Medicum in Stockholm had the rights to bodies of suicide victims and children born out of wedlock.[17] These were the same persons who were denied Christian burial, which implies that dissection was understood to be a desecration or a retribution to which the bodies of honest citizens would not be subjected.

Nine years later, the Collegium Medicum was also granted rights to the corpses of persons who had died at various correctional institutions (those under arrest or in spinning houses or penitentiaries), hospitals, and poorhouses. This could have meant a significant increase in the number of bodies available. However, when Algot Key-Åberg, professor of forensic medicine and medical jurisprudence at the Karolinska Institute, commented on this availability in his 1889 compilation of historical regulation of dissection corpses for the medical schools in Stockholm, Uppsala, and Lund, he maintained that "it has never been possible, except perhaps during the time just after [the law's] enactment, to act upon this right to any significant degree, and that quite soon, probably mainly due to an oppositional general public opinion, [it] must be as good as given up entirely."[18]

In an 1814 letter to His Royal Majesty, the Sundhetskollegiet (Sweden's College of Health) requested access to more bodies for anatomical instruction through more accommodating regulations. However, the results were not what the doctors had hoped. Deferring to "the gravity of the matter" and the prejudices of the lower classes, the government decided instead to limit bodies for dissection to three types. First were the criminals, who were considered to have "forfeited civil freedom" by committing crimes. Second and third were the institutionalized poor and the mentally ill whose survivors could not afford to pay funeral expenses, if they had *also* been indecent and depraved. Prisons, workhouses, and asylums were legally bound to report the deaths of individuals who might be considered anatomical objects, but these laws were not always followed. Many corpses were thus never delivered to the medical schools, which points to a likely hidden conflict between anatomists and those who ran the institutions for the poor and mentally ill.[19]

Because of public resistance, medical institutions could not in practice obtain all of the corpses to which they had rights. According to Key-Åberg, in 1889 anatomists had access to

> (1) dead, specially-qualified prisoners and wards of the state from workhouses and general institutions for the care of the poor operated by the city of Stockholm . . . as well as 2) possibly, individuals not residing in the municipality of Stockholm, who have died at such institutions, and who have neither the means to cover funeral costs nor family members who will see to their burial.
>
> In addition, access to the dead bodies of illegitimate children, in those cases where no hindrances exist, should in actuality depend upon whether or not the child's mother or nearest relatives create obstacles to the use of such a corpse for the purposes of anatomical study.[20]

To obtain access to corpses, university medical departments had to submit requisitions for the number of corpses they needed one by one, whereupon it was the responsibility of the police to see to transport.

What emerges from contemporary reports, laws, and regulations is a picture of wide-ranging activity involving corpses. In poorhouses, hospitals, and prisons, the dead were laid in coffins or stuffed into simple containers, which were then transported by wagon, train, or steamboat. A law from 1884 stated that if these crates were sent over long distances, they must be marked with the word "naturalia."[21] The documents accompanying the corpses were to be stamped by railway personnel and the police. When the crates arrived at the medical schools, they were received by the custodian and stored in a cool place, ready to be unpacked, embalmed, and dissected. Finally, the remains were buried after dissection. Many people, not just doctors, were thus involved in this traffic of dead bodies. The strictness of the laws and regulations indicates that legislators thought it was important for corpses to be handled in a secure and efficient manner.

While legislators went to great lengths to satisfy the anatomists, there was, in fact, a tug-of-war between doctors and lawmakers. Again and again in their reports, doctors complained about a shortage of corpses. The state, however, tried to balance the doctors' demands against the need to be sensitive to public opinion. What the doctors dismissed as the superstition of the uneducated poor, the government had to respect when regulating issues concerning dead body materials (where they should be obtained and similar points). In general, the government was very accommodating and gave the Karolinska Institute, for example, all the funding it needed to expand and improve this work.[22]

In principle, the regulations passed between 1814 and 1932 contained nothing new.[23] The rules from 1814 remained in effect, although additions were made over time. The number of institutions affected by these rules grew continually, as did the number of corpses made available to medical schools. Each change occurred after pressure from university anatomy departments. In 1880, His Royal Majesty allowed the Karolinska Institute and the medical faculty at Uppsala University access to deceased prisoners from the entire country of Sweden, except the province of Skåne where Lund University was situated. Earlier, the government declared that Stockholm and Uppsala were to share a smaller area; this update gave them a welcome increase.[24] Institutions other than medical departments also wanted rights to dead bodies: in 1880, Stockholm's Gymnastiska centralinstitut (the Institute of Gymnastics and Physiotherapy) was granted the right to three corpses per year, and the Royal Academy of Fine Arts received rights to one. In the case of fine arts students, the instructor was to select a suitable corpse; academic ideals placed aesthetic requirements on the dead models.[25]

Departments of anatomy were also granted increased corpse quotas through new permissions for the transfer of dead bodies. Previously, such transfer had only been permitted during the coolest months of the year. In 1881, transfers were also permitted during the month of May, and in 1888 this policy was increased to include the entire year, on the condition that the corpses were not stored more than forty-eight hours in mortuaries or cellars during the warm months.[26] Improved methods for cold storage lay behind this new regulation. A number of temporary rules were introduced in 1926. These were based on existing regulations but contained some innovations. The family of the deceased was given the right to require a normal burial, even if they were unable to pay for it, and they were allowed five days to submit their request, as opposed to the previous three. The revised rules also expressly stated that after its use for anatomical purposes, the corpse should be given a dignified burial. Earlier regulations had merely stipulated a "suitable" burial.[27]

Effective January 1, 1933, all of the old regulations were replaced by a new civil code that to a large extent remained in effect until 1973. This law was stricter: the three-day limit returned, and if they were unable to pay for the funeral, family members could no longer influence the fate of the deceased's body.[28] Much of this new law was similar to older legislation. It was still the responsibility of the police to report the deaths of suitable persons and to send their bodies to the proper anatomy department. The only such departments were still those in Lund, Uppsala, and Stockholm; and it was still the responsibility of the Karolinska Institute to distribute three corpses per year to Stockholm's Institute of Gymnastics and Physiotherapy and one to the Royal Academy of Fine Arts.[29] The new code also expressly stated that the corpse should be given a funeral and burial.

One of the new provisions in the 1933 law was that the only corpses that could be claimed for anatomical purposes would be those that otherwise would have to be buried at public expense, regardless of the background of the deceased and regardless of where or at which institution the individual had died. Exempt from being used for anatomical purposes were corpses the family could take care of, those that were carriers of contagious diseases, those that needed to be examined for forensic purposes, and those that had become unusable as a result of some "extreme transformation."[30] Interestingly, the legislators were still respectful of public opinion: "The transport of corpses shall be undertaken by the most inexpensive means, without disregard for the respect which should be shown and which is demanded by the general public, and shall be paid for by the department of anatomy to which the corpse is delivered."[31]

There was no change in the traditional legislation concerning the use of corpses for anatomical purposes until 1973, when a donation system was introduced. Beginning that year, an entirely new way of thinking came into effect, in which an individual could decide whether his or her body would be left to science after death. Previously, the individual's autonomy and opinion on the matter were entirely subordinate to the interests of science. This change reflected a profound change in sensibilities and ethical standards. There were also practical reasons why the change in Swedish law was passed at that point in time: the World Health Organization (WHO) had recommended that all its member nations change their legislation in that direction, and it had become difficult for anatomy departments to obtain a sufficient number of corpses under the old regulations.[32]

Clinical Autopsies

During the second half of the nineteenth century in Sweden, the terms *obduktion* and *autopsi* were used interchangeably.[33] The Latin word *obducere* actually means "to close" or "to put back into place," emphasizing, oddly enough, the conclusion of this activity. The word *autopsy* stems from the

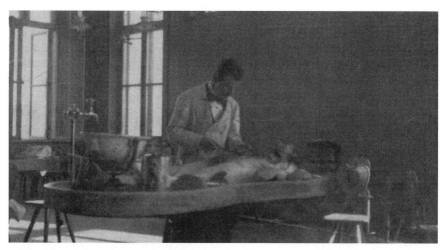

Figure 3. Early-twentieth-century autopsy, Department of Pathological Anatomy, Karolinska Institute. From Israel Holmgren, *Mitt liv* (Stockholm, 1959), plate 21. Duplication: Kungl. biblioteket - National Library of Sweden.

Greek language and points more to the work itself: roughly, it means "to see with one's own eyes."[34]

In a clinical autopsy, the parts of the body are studied very carefully to identify changes in organs and tissues caused by disease or injury. Autopsies are conducted for many reasons, among which discovering the cause of death is only one. An autopsy can also provide answers to questions of how a medical treatment affected the body, and it allows comparisons with diagnoses made when the patient was alive.[35]

The principles for conducting an autopsy are the same today as they were around the turn of the twentieth century. The doctor, a pathologist, often has the help of assistants during the procedure. Together, they conduct and record the autopsy, which begins with a visual inspection of the exterior of the corpse. Then, knives, saws, and scissors are used to open the body cavities—that is, the chest, abdomen, and skull. The organs are removed, taken apart, and cut into sections. Tissues that exhibit changes as a result of disease are often examined under a microscope or by chemical means. Sometimes certain body parts are stored and preserved for further analysis. The doctor studies the shape, color, size, and texture of the organs. When the examination is complete, the organs are put back into the body, and it is sewn shut. The goal is for family members who pay their final respects to be unable to see that the body has been subjected to an autopsy.

In his 1959 autobiography, physician Israel Holmgren published a photograph taken in the autopsy room of the Karolinska Institute in the early early twentieth century (see figure 3).[36] The photograph provides an idea

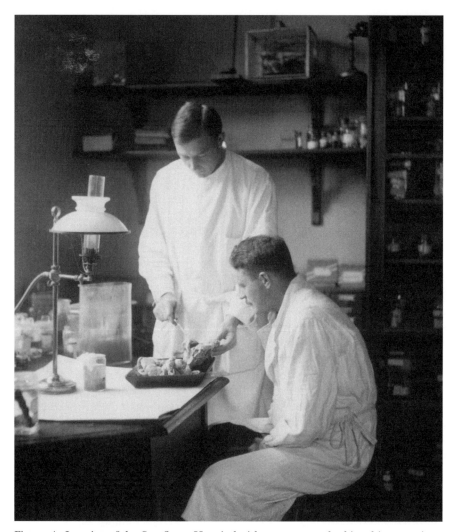

Figure 4. Interior of the Serafimer Hospital with two men garbed in white examining a specimen and with glass jars containing chemicals and specimens on the tables and shelves. Photograph by Axel Malmström (undated, circa 1910). Stockholm City Museum.

of working conditions for doctors and medical students. Illumination was still provided by gas lamps, and protective gloves had not yet been introduced.[37] In another photograph from Serafimer Hospital in Stockholm, two men in white lab clothing are seen examining a cutout body part (see figure 4). The desk before them is covered with glass jars of various sizes, containing preparations and preservative fluids. The shelf behind them is also lined with jars full of specimens. The picture is not dated, and the men are unnamed, but the photo was probably taken around 1900. The men are likely studying something that had been obtained through a clinical autopsy at the hospital.

Just as the number of anatomical dissections increased during the nineteenth century, so did the number of clinical autopsies as a result of the increased importance of pathology in medicine. Clinical autopsies were conducted at various health care facilities (such as hospitals, clinics, asylums), where they were regulated by the laws governing Swedish hospitals. They were also conducted at pathology institutions and sometimes in milieus not suited to this work, such as sheds and even homes.[38]

An autopsy is similar in nature to an anatomical dissection (even though autopsies were less stigmatizing, since they were often performed on corpses of members of the upper class—kings, professors, and their peers—whereas dissection cadavers were deceased poor people). It is therefore not surprising that the general public also found autopsies transgressive. Given physicians' great interest in pathology, it is also not surprising that conflicts arose concerning the work of pathologists as well.

On April 21, 1874, Professor Axel Key referred to such a conflict in a lecture to the Swedish Society of Medicine that dealt with the case of a seventeen-year-old boy who had died at the hospital in the town of Värnamo on April 3 of that year. A piece of the boy's spinal cord had been removed during an autopsy, preserved, and sent to Key by a Dr. Nordenström. The spinal cord was afflicted by both cancer and scurvy and was regarded as an interesting pathological specimen. Key described the specimen carefully and compared it with the case description and autopsy report sent in by Nordenström. It was a typical pathology lecture for the time. Especially interesting is a parenthetical note that interrupts Dr. Nordenström's report on the autopsy: "The examination of the brain was now to be undertaken, but was hindered by the arrival of the family of the deceased, who had never actually given permission for the autopsy, and who now prevented its continuation."[39]

It is easy to imagine the dismay the parents felt when they learned what was being done with their son's body. Opening the head is a particularly sensitive procedure: the skin of the face has to be peeled back, and the thick skull bone has to be opened with a saw. How did they prevent the autopsy from continuing? Was there a scuffle? Regardless of what actually took place, the quotation merits closer examination. The family had *never actually given permission for the autopsy*—indicating that the doctor had either known the family's wishes and consciously gone against them or that the hospital had never asked about the family's feelings. For the doctor conducting the autopsy, it was clearly annoying that the procedure had to be stopped halfway through. The quotation carries more of a tone of apology to the doctor's colleagues than one of regret that the family had been upset. Further, nothing is said about whether the family had given permission for a piece of the boy's spinal tissue to be removed and preserved outside his body. Those who opposed the autopsy would probably not have wanted his body to be cut up this way, but the issue is avoided through silence.

Clearly, this is a scientific lecture about a sarcoma of the spinal column and not a talk about the seventeen-year-old boy and his family. Nonetheless, the sentence quoted here opens perspective, providing a glimpse of the fundamental differences between the views about dead bodies held by pathologists compared with the lay public. What for the pathologist was a scientific object that might possibly add to his reputation if it demonstrated something unusual was something altogether different for the family.

This scenario is not unique. Similar situations are hinted at in many case descriptions, such as those in the papers of the Swedish Society of Medicine. However, conflicts of this type are difficult to identify or find material about—they can only be glimpsed in occasional phrases and parentheses. Sometimes, we can see that a doctor has accommodated the survivors' wishes, as in a case description from 1894 in which the doctor wrote that "out of respect for the wishes of the family, [he] opened . . . only the abdominal cavity."[40] Further, I have found no traces of conflicts concerning autopsied bodies in the form of legal proceedings. This may result from the fact that the practice of clinical autopsies was not regulated by law and that poor people had no means to pursue legal processes.

Legislation Concerning Autopsies

Clinical autopsies were regulated only by local rules and statutes. Thus, for example, the mission statement of Allmänna försörjningsinrättningen (General Poorhouse) in Stockholm, written November 16, 1865, declared that a doctor there should, "when such is *deemed by him to be necessary,* undertake an autopsy upon a patient who has died in this institution, and shall keep a record of the examination in a special book."[41] In 1870, when the General Poorhouse was included among the institutions that were to provide corpses for anatomical dissection, the law emphasized that autopsy work could not be jeopardized. Autopsies were deemed more important than dissections, and departments of anatomy were actually only given access to the bodies of destitute persons not judged to require an autopsy.[42]

In 1875, a rule was introduced for students of the Karolinska Institute doing internships at "those medical institutions related to it," that is, Serafimer Hospital, the General Maternity Hospital, and Garrison Hospital.[43] The interns were now *required* to participate in autopsies, especially those conducted on patients about whom they had kept notes. This rule indicates the importance of the anatomo-clinical method: medical students were expected to acquire pathological experience by comparing autopsy results to the diagnoses and treatments made while the patients were alive. The students were also required to learn how to prepare an autopsy report under their teachers' supervision.[44]

In 1901, a general law for Sweden's hospitals was passed, in which physicians were charged

> to, insofar as no cases of medical jurisprudence may be involved, undertake autopsies upon patients who have died at the hospital, when the cause of death is unknown or an important insight into the nature of the disease may be achieved. *If the family desires that an autopsy shall not be performed, then such shall be performed only in those cases in which the cause of death is unknown.* In cases in which an examination for the purpose of medical jurisprudence enters into question, the physician shall immediately submit an application to the proper authority, which shall, if such an examination is found necessary, appoint another physician.[45]

In this context, the statement that it is the physician's *responsibility* to undertake an autopsy may indicate that not all hospital physicians were interested in conducting autopsies. Pathologists and the National Board of Medicine wanted to compile death statistics, a process facilitated by this law. Individual doctors, on the other hand, might have preferred not to cut into their patients' dead bodies. One can imagine that a doctor in a small, rural town who was close to his patients would have been more reluctant to conduct autopsies than pathologists in a university clinic. It could be difficult to defend an autopsy before surviving relatives who regarded the procedure as disrespectful of the deceased. In addition, autopsies could reveal faulty diagnoses and treatments gone wrong, something not all doctors would want to make public.

The hierarchical order of prioritization among the different dissection-related activities is also worth noting: forensic autopsies had the highest priority, followed by clinical autopsies and, finally, anatomical dissections. The interests of society thus weighed more heavily than clinical ones, and educational interests were of still lesser importance. Scientific interests ended up in a sort of intermediate position between clinical and anatomical ones. Yet even though scientific interests did not hold a strong position within the law, doctors collected clinical material for scientific purposes (as exemplified by Axel Key's speech to the Swedish Society of Medicine, mentioned earlier).

The basic components of Sweden's 1901 law remained in effect throughout most of the twentieth century and can be seen in health care legislation as late as 1972. A new law regarding autopsies came into effect in 1976, in which a new rule was introduced: if the deceased had not given written consent for an autopsy, the surviving relatives were to be informed before the

autopsy could be conducted.[46] Until as recently as 1976, it was not considered important that the relatives even know what was to be done with a dead
person's body, and the possibilities for them to influence those activities
were thus limited. The interests of society were given priority before those of
the individual, and knowledge received priority over autonomy, as was also
the case with anatomical dissections.

Forensic Autopsies

The difference between a forensic and a clinical autopsy is determined by
the different questions posed during the examination. A forensic examination is performed when there is suspicion that the deceased was the victim
of a crime or in the case of unexpected, difficult-to-explain deaths. The
purpose of a forensic autopsy also means that the methods used differ to
some extent from those used in a clinical autopsy. Much greater emphasis is
placed on the examination of the exterior of the body, and chemical analysis
is used to identify substances such as poisons.

Although the technical methods available at the turn of the twentieth
century seem very limited by today's standards, crimes could in many cases
be identified or solved. This can be seen clearly in the collection of autopsy
reports published in 1916 by Algot Key-Åberg.[47] The reports follow a standardized format and always begin with the date of the autopsy, the names
of both the deceased and the person writing the report, and several items
of a formal nature, followed by a brief summary of the police report on the
events surrounding the incidence of death. After this introductory information, the actual autopsy report begins.

The heading "Exterior Examination" is almost always followed by the
statement "the body lies naked upon the dissection table." The minute
details of the exterior examination are reported according to a predetermined procedure. The interior examination begins with of the underside
of the scalp and continues through all the body's organs, tissues, and fluids.
The reports use colorful, descriptive language and are more detailed when
anything unusual or remarkable is encountered. This example deals with a
lung belonging to a four-month-old baby boy who, according to the report,
probably died of acute pneumonia:

> The surface is marbled in flecks, with generally larger brown-violet sections
> and smaller gray-red ones, the latter of which have risen above the former. The
> pleura is smooth and shiny. . . . The cross-section, also marbled with darker
> and lighter sections, is overall even and moist, and is in some spots more and
> some spots less obviously porous.[48]

The report concludes with a statement in which the physician summarizes the autopsy and presents points that may have bearing on the crime investigation and whether a crime may be suspected.

Strikingly, many of the examples in Key-Åberg's collection deal with women who died as a result of failed attempts at illegal abortions, as well as with fetuses or newborn babies suspected to have been murdered. The fact that crimes of this type were common gives us insight into a society that offered grim alternatives for women who experienced unwanted pregnancies. It also highlights the fact that the working conditions of forensic scientists have changed over the course of history: social changes bring changes in the nature of crimes and thus in the types of injuries seen on the autopsy table. The same tendency can be seen in the *Rättsmedicinsk atlas* (*Atlas of Legal Medicine*) from 1898.[49] A disproportionately large section is devoted to close-up photographs of female genitalia (fifty-seven photographs, compared with four photographs of male genitalia). This simply cannot be explained by pedagogical needs. Even within forensic medicine, evidence exists of the obsessive study of female sexuality that was at the center of nineteenth-century medical science.[50]

Legislation Concerning Forensic Science

While clinical autopsies were less strictly regulated than anatomical dissections, the opposite was true for examinations of bodily injuries caused by crime. The discipline of forensic medicine was established in the eighteenth century, but even early on regulations were in place requiring an examination of dead bodies when a crime was suspected.[51] In Sweden, such examinations were required to be made by a physician, according to a 1770 royal decree. Prior to this, the task had fallen to laymen, often members of the local district council. In the beginning of the 1800s, regulations regarding medicolegal examinations and autopsies were developed by the College of Health. In 1818, these regulations were given the status of law.[52]

In 1886, two new laws replaced the 1818 legislation. The first of these laid forth detailed regulations for the practical, legal, and bureaucratic circumstances surrounding the opening of dead bodies, as well as matters of responsibility, reporting, decision making, and similar issues. This law also established that a forensic autopsy must consist of two parts: an examination of the exterior of the body, followed by the opening of the body. It also stated that the doctor should "take pains that the opened body, at the conclusion of the autopsy, shall be closed up in a suitable manner."[53]

The second law consisted of rules developed by the National Board of Medicine as to how a forensic examination should proceed. These rules are very detailed and cover everything from which instruments a doctor should carry to how a cut should be made and how lesions should be observed.[54]

The degree of detail in the regulations may seem surprising, especially in comparison with the regulations for clinical autopsies and anatomical dissections, which contain no details about how the procedures should be conducted. The reason, of course, is the altogether different nature of forensic medicine, where the doctor is working within the sphere of jurisprudence. For the results to be satisfactory and usable in such contexts, the methods used must be transparent and identical for each individual case. In regard to autopsies conducted for purely scientific reasons, doctors have to answer only to each other, while forensic activity must be understandable to, and reliable for, persons without medical knowledge (e.g., policemen, lawyers, judges). The Medical Board's meticulous rules were also intended to guarantee the quality of autopsies even in rural areas, where educated doctors were not always available.

The need for forensic autopsies was easily justified, and we might expect that the general public found them easier to accept than those undertaken primarily for the sake of science. The family of someone believed to have been murdered should have been interested to see that justice was done (assuming they were not themselves guilty). Yet even in forensic contexts, we find a resistance to the opening of dead bodies, which can be illustrated by a legal case in the city of Gävle that attracted public attention.

In 1896, Pastor Johan Petrus Norberg, a leader of the Mission Covenant Church of Sweden, was accused of murdering his housemaid, Johanna Charlotta Lennström. For some time, the housemaid had suffered from a difficult condition that afflicted her in the form of spastic attacks. The doctors were not sure whether the attacks were caused by epilepsy, hysteria, or something else altogether. Her death was followed by a comprehensive forensic examination in which the experts reached differing conclusions. The case was also debated in the press. Was Norberg guilty? In an attempt to clear his name, Norberg published his own account of the events surrounding the death. He claimed he had done everything he could to save his housemaid when she had an attack but that in the end she had fallen and struck her head on a stone in the woods and could not be saved.[55]

In the debate over the case, details from the forensic examination were publicized in the daily newspapers and discussed openly. Talking about such subjects was not taboo, and it was also not unusual for newspapers to discuss suicides in detail. The problem lay not at that level of discourse but instead in the public's emotional resistance to the autopsy. In the Norberg case, the housemaid's sisters were opposed to the autopsy, despite the fact that a doctor had tried to convince them of its necessity.[56] In the court protocol, the sisters' opposition to the autopsy was interpreted as a "very common occurrence, since many find autopsy especially repugnant to the senses and a disturbance of the peace of the dead."[57]

However, when the case became a police matter, the autopsy could be undertaken without the family's consent, which outraged the sisters. Norberg described the events:

> Toward the evening, the older sister of the deceased came running to me, and in tears told me that she had heard that through the authority of the police, an autopsy was already under way at the crypt under the direction of Dr. Åman, and she asked whether we knew of this. We had heard nothing about it, and I found it difficult to believe this report, since not even the family of the deceased had been informed. Yet upon making inquiries we found that it was so, as she had heard. She was most painfully moved by this report, and found it difficult that she had not been deemed worthy to be properly informed of this matter, which concerned her so closely.[58]

Norberg claimed that he himself had no objections to the autopsy and that he would have gladly witnessed it if he had been allowed to do so. Does this indicate that attitudes toward autopsies were a matter of social class? It is possible that a member of the educated middle class, such as Norberg, found it easier to accept the benefits of an autopsy than the housemaid's family did. However, Norberg's positive stance toward the autopsy was also necessary in this situation, as it was important for him to appear to be an innocent man who had nothing to hide.

Modernity, Power, and the Body

The attitudes of medical scientists toward the body, and the use of corpses as objects of research and education, were certainly not commonplace or generally accepted among the public. In her book *Death, Dissection, and the Destitute*, British medical historian Ruth Richardson discusses the emotional and symbolic meanings dissection held for anatomists. Anatomical dissection, according to Richardson, requires that the practitioner shut off or put aside normal physical and emotional reactions to the act, which involves willfully mutilating the body of another human being. "It requires working 'beyond the range of ordinary emotions.' "[59] Practice is needed to complete the work and to achieve a detached attitude, which the famous eighteenth-century anatomist William Hunter called "a kind of necessary inhumanity."

In this context, anatomy courses for medical students, with their obligatory dissections, function as a rite of initiation: the dissections are of decisive importance for the doctor-to-be to acquire the expected detached attitude. Detachment and a rational view are necessary for doctors to uphold their legitimacy.[60] The professional distancing also means anatomists, pathologists, and forensic doctors are given a special status in Western culture, in which the corpse is surrounded by strict cultural rules—the corpse is not to be touched, other than in certain ritual acts and during the measures that must be taken between death and burial. This section examines the medical profession's positive attitude, as well as the general public's repulsion, toward the opening of dead bodies. These attitudes will be considered in relation to legislation, modernity, and power.

General Repulsion toward the Opening of Dead Bodies

An important element in the opposition to autopsies is distaste for opening the body. Cutting into the dead was seen as a violent and transgressive act. The survivors felt the dead body should be preserved intact. What is the background for this notion?

The simplest explanation is that Christian tradition maintained that the bodies of the dead must be preserved intact to rise up again on judgment day. Yet people knew that corpses decayed in the grave, that they broke down and lost their shape, so this explanation is insufficient. Religious ideas do, however, provide part of the context. The belief within the great monotheistic religions that human beings are made in the image of God means that intrusions into the (dead) body are often seen as violations of both the human being and of God. Literal belief in the physical resurrection of the dead may be uncommon in modern Protestantism, but, Christianity consists not only of theology but also of incorporated folk traditions and rituals. Within this realm of ideas, conceptions of a bodily resurrection may be important.[61]

Religious ideas could also be combined with magical ones. Folklorist Louise Hagberg has shown that it was important for amputated limbs and even wigs to be placed in the grave with the deceased. But was this done so the dead would be intact at resurrection? No, it was done so they would not walk the earth. According to Swedish folk belief, a dead person who was missing a body part would not find peace until it was found, and human bones could also be used as amulets and tools for performing magic.[62] Ideas such as these could apparently be applied to bodies subjected to autopsies or dissections. Bodies stored in outbuildings and corpse sheds while awaiting burial were treated with terrified reverence. Bodies were to be handled with respect. The places where they were kept were surrounded by mystery and horror stories. Those who handled, washed, and enshrouded corpses also had a special status in society, examined in more detail in chapter 4.

The opening of a dead body for medical purposes is fundamentally different from the traditional ways of caring for, washing, and enshrouding corpses, and it is little wonder that it was perceived as a disrespectful act. Widespread distrust of medical doctors and their activities in general contributed to the public's skepticism.[63] The power of and respect for the dead in tradition and custom, together with a general dislike of doctors, formed

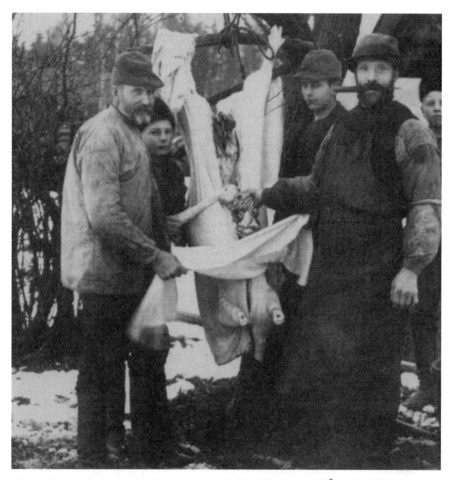

Figure 5. Butcher A. E. Alm slaughtering a pig in the town of Örebro, 1898. Photograph by Sam Lindskog. From, "Sam Lindskog, Kgl. Hoffotograf, Örebro," *Från bergslag och bondebygd 1983*, ed. Egon Thun (Örebro Läns Museum, Sweden: 1983), 25. Duplication: Kungl. biblioteket - National Library of Sweden.

a basis for the reluctance to turn over dead friends and relatives for a treatment as unusual as dissection.

A further aspect of the abhorrence to opening dead bodies is its similarity to the slaughter of animals. Slaughtering was something everyone who lived in the country, and even many in the cities, were familiar with in the days before large, centralized slaughterhouses. In an 1898 photograph from Örebro, the headless, gutted body of a pig hangs upside down from a tree branch, surrounded by two grown men and three boys (see figure 5). The man with the beard, hat, and apron is the butcher. He is posing with a knife in his mouth and entrails in one hand. The presence of the children indicates the everyday nature of the situation. The similarity of slaughter to dissection and autopsy becomes clear when considered this way, even more so for those who have witnessed the slaughter of animals: both activities deal with cutting up bodies and dividing them into various parts. It is not difficult to imagine that people could feel revulsion toward having the bodies of their dead relatives cut up like pigs at slaughter or that anatomists and autopsy doctors were skeptically regarded as a sort of butcher or executioner. In the common understanding, there are great similarities between the activities of the autopsy doctor and the butcher, although human bodies are granted the honor of a funeral and farm animals are not.

Anatomy as Punishment

Another aspect of this matter involves methods of punishment. In earlier eras, a sentence could be made more severe by imposing further punishments on the body of an executed criminal: beheaded criminals could also be burned; those who had been hung might be left out to be eaten by birds; the body could be mutilated and parts of it nailed up in public view.[64] When anatomists began to make use of the bodies of executed criminals, the consideration of dissection as a severe punishment or a sort of mutilation soon followed. In his article "Frithiof Holmgren och straffanatomin" ("Frithiof Holmgren and Anatomy as Penalty"), historian Torbjörn Gustafsson describes how anatomists took up a position within the Swedish legal system as a form of extra-executioners who tortured dead bodies. With a background in physiology, Holmgren regarded the executed criminal on the dissection table as a type of martyr who had been sacrificed to science.[65]

Gustafsson and others use the expression "anatomy as punishment" as a matter of course—it seems an accepted fact that anatomical dissection was used as and understood to be a punishment.[66] How did this come to be? The thought that a body could be punished further after death is rather remarkable, yet it is rooted in old ideas. The border between life and death was poorly defined and changeable. A sort of "afterlife" was tied to the dead body, and the courts could sentence bodies to various punishments, including the death penalty. Into the eighteenth century, if a criminal or his or her dead body could not be produced, a substitute body in the form of a picture or an effigy could be penalized in its place.[67] Nineteenth-century legal texts concerning anatomy emphasized the terrifying effect anatomy had on the living. This terror may have been tied to beliefs that the body continued to be alive in some sense even after death and that the dead could suffer.

The old laws that regulated anatomical and pathological activity attest to a view of human life that seems foreign in our era. Anatomical dissection was held to be a terrifying punishment outside the established penal code. Indecent and depraved inmates of poorhouses and hospitals who died were sent to anatomists—an "expedient correction for the poor," according to an 1814 royal decree.[68] In this context, citizens seem primarily to have been objects for the moralistic exercise of power yet also economic objects, in the sense that those without means were made to provide a final service to the state to justify their burial.

A few lines from the 1814 ordinance show, however, that authorities were conscious of the risk of taking this too far:

> [W]ere the parish poorhouses subjected to so extreme an arrangement as has been suggested by the College of Health for the amelioration of the shortages in anatomical education, it would undoubtedly result in mistrust and aversion on the part of the poorer members of the populace, who would thwart and weaken the diligence and progress of the poorhouse boards, as well as general trust and charity, such that the important goals of the poorhouses would to a significant degree be hampered and ineffective.[69]

In Great Britain, the 1832 anatomy law, which granted anatomists the right to obtain the corpses of all those who had died in institutions that cared for the poor, further strengthened the shame associated with poorhouses. By holding lavish funerals, the poor did everything they could to prove that their loved ones had not died at the expense of the public and thus had escaped the dissection knife.[70]

In Swedish laws, it is difficult to discern exactly which corpses could be legally turned over to anatomists and even more difficult to find out which ones actually were provided to them. It is certain that until 1973, only people with a very weak position in society were thus affected. Depending upon the perspective from which the question is asked, somewhat different variations of the same theme emerge. In a 1986 essay on legal history, Göran Inger identified one of the tendencies of the state: the bodies that were turned over to anatomists were those of people who, during life, had through their own actions placed themselves outside society, those who "were deemed to have lost their honor, decency and personal worth."[71] Sweden's 1992 commission on organ transplants emphasized the economic aspect: "The right to a dead body was less a question of personal integrity than [of] purely economic convenience."[72] If the issue is viewed from the perspective of power and gender, as exemplified by Karin Johannisson, the conclusion is that at the very end of life, already marginalized and stigmatized individuals, such as gypsies and prostitutes, were degraded and robbed of their humanity by men of power.[73]

The earliest laws gave anatomists the right to procure the corpses of executed criminals, derelicts, and illegitimate children. Thus the objects of anatomy came to be linked with crime, sin, and shame. It is true that these unfortunates received a decent burial after their dissections were completed; otherwise, they would have been buried outside the consecrated ground of the cemetery, symbolically placing them outside society even after death. The dead were deemed to have atoned for their sins because their bodies had served science and thus finally been of benefit to humanity.

Yet judging from the common public aversion, which anatomists maintained was based on superstition, the fate of dissection was considered worse than that of an ignominious burial. The characterization of dissection as a punishment continued and was strengthened by the ordinance that granted anatomists the right to the corpses of those who had died at public expense in poorhouses and penal institutions and who were furthermore considered indecent and lewd. In 1932, this law's link to crime was broken, but its connection to poverty continued in Sweden until 1973, when the donation system was introduced.

Prior to 1973, legislation concerning anatomy placed the bodies of the dead within an economic and moralistic framework, in which benefits to science were central—a form of utilitarian thinking that during the second half of the twentieth century fell out of step with the times (at least in regard to this issue) and was replaced by an emphasis on individual autonomy and the power of determination over one's own body.

The Body, Beneficial and Grotesque

Even doctors seem to have viewed dissection as a less-than-suitable fate for a dead human being, at least when their own bodies were in question. The majority of doctors were unwilling to donate their brains when Gustaf Retzius and Robert Tigerstedt tried to organize a "brain club" for the study of "elite brains" in the late 1880s.[74] During the nineteenth century, attempts were made to change the negative attitude toward scientific intrusions into the body after death. Utilitarian philosopher Jeremy Bentham arranged for his body to be preserved and displayed after his death and donated this "Auto Icon" to London University College in the belief that he was providing a good example.[75] Doctors and scientists considered it important for people to realize a corpse's scientific and thus social value. Reason was to take precedence over emotion, and the greater good was considered more important than minor evils.

When Erik Müller became professor of anatomy at the Karolinska Institute in 1899, he stated in his inaugural lecture that death was made beneficial by the study of anatomy. He drew a dark picture of the past, in which his colleagues had to endure hardships because of the negative attitudes of the general populace. From his perspective, though, conditions had improved:

Of Vesalius and his contemporaries, it is related that they were often reduced to satisfying their research needs in cemeteries and places of execution. Even into the seventeenth and the beginning of the eighteenth century, anatomists complained about the ill-will directed from the lower levels of society toward those who occupied themselves with the study of corpses. Dark, secluded cellars were often the only refuges where "death could delight in saving life."[76]

This is a classic story of progress, of the evolution of science, of a heroic professional group that had to battle a superstitious populace. Müller and his colleagues associated "the study of corpses" with enlightenment and social benefit. For Müller, the individual, hands-on dissection training for medical students introduced during the nineteenth century was a decisive improvement in medical education. Dissections provided doctors-to-be with a "living image" of the interior of a human being, something the students would carry with them for the rest of their lives. Dissections would also "teach [students] the difficult art of observation" and allow them to develop dexterity.[77]

At the dedication of the new dissection hall at Uppsala in 1884, anatomy professor Edvard Clason gave a speech in which he emphasized similar positive aspects of the practice of dissection. However, Clason also stressed another theme: he challenged the students to attain inner and outer purity. He was aware that anatomists' work could be perceived as distasteful, and he charged the students to take no notice: "We must work with many things that according to the common understanding are loathsome and filthy, yet let us do so in a way that our innermost [self] is not thereby defiled."[78]

Clason also understood that doctors could be regarded as (philosophical) materialists or even cynical and that they were "regarded as having acquired this view of life during their student years and especially in the anatomy laboratory." Clason countered this accusation by maintaining that the work in a dissection hall should induce serious thoughts and have a humbling and purifying effect, for several reasons. First and foremost, the dissection hall on a daily basis revealed the highest organism in creation as it appeared when exposed to forces of decay. Second, this was a place where death was conquered, since "through its crimes it must serve life." Third, the work material, which consisted of "the maimed limbs of unfortunate fellow human beings," should produce feelings of compassion.[79] Clason denied emphatically that anatomists should distance themselves or become inhumane, as Hunter had claimed.[80]

Outer purity was closely tied to inner purity: "We desire tidy specimens in this new hall, as well as tidiness in the hall and tidy dissectors." It was important that this purity was applied to more than just mental hygiene. Although the corpses prepared for dissection had been embalmed with disinfectant liquids, those slated for autopsy might be contagious. Bodies were opened without protective gloves, and it was important to clean one's sores to avoid being infected by "corpse poisons." Strict order was necessary to maintain the health of the body as well as of the soul. The old dissection hall had been far too crowded to keep clean, but a new day was dawning.[81]

Why this need to maintain inner purity and to banish "raw, cynical joking" from the dissection hall? Clearly, a problem was being concealed. Dead bodies, slashed corpses, are provocative, and order must be maintained if they are to be dealt with. Stories of the desecration of bodies by anatomy students are also numerous.[82]

Not all these stories are myths. Rough pranks took place in anatomy halls, as proven by a series of photographs from the early 1900s, preserved at the Medical Museion in Copenhagen. (The photos are unique for Scandinavia but common in the United States.[83] The pictures are so graphic that it is easy to understand why similar photographs have often been discarded from other collections.) One of the photos shows a number of men, most in white overcoats and one wearing a hat (see figure 6). One of them busies himself with the lower leg of a cadaver. In the center of the picture, a skeleton stands dressed as a dissector, with a white overcoat, cigarette in its mouth, a saw in one hand, and gesturing like a teacher. Perhaps this was a harmless student joke, but it was not respectful and "pure" behavior in Clason's ideal view. Another photograph is more grotesque (see figure 7). In the room are six men and three women. A skeleton stands in the center of this photograph as well, embracing two of the women. Two cadavers are laid out on dissection tables; the one on the right is propped up with its spread-open posterior facing the camera. A man fingers a severed head while another stands beside him, grinning. A light-hearted mood clearly fills the room.

In *Presence in the Flesh: The Body in Medicine,* anthropologist Katharine Young observes the grotesque nature of the dissected body. She suggests that it has characteristics of the carnival grotesquery studied by Mikhail Bakhtin. The grotesque, Bakhtin wrote, ignores the boundaries and surfaces of the body. The grotesque image of the body shows not only the exterior but also its interior, consisting of blood, entrails, and other organs. The interior and exterior are merged.[84] Dissection dissolves the separation between the body and the surrounding world and breaks down the body's normal form; it divides it into parts, destroys its order, and makes it grotesque.[85] The carnival atmosphere is signified by the upside down or inside out, the transgression of borders, mutilation, and associations with entrails and feces, slaughter and pigs.

At the end of the seventeenth century, when dissection retreated from the gaze of the paying public and increasingly became an exclusive element of medicine, it was, according to Young, an attempt to present anatomy as pure, refined, and "aristocratic."[86] To preserve the hierarchical exclusivity of discourse, the grotesque body must be concealed. In this way, the grotesque body of the anatomical sciences became a threat to medical discourse.

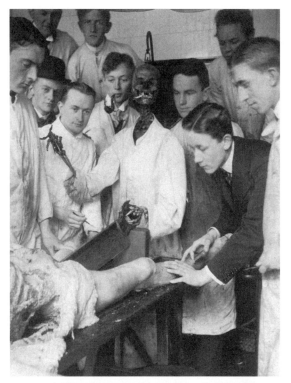

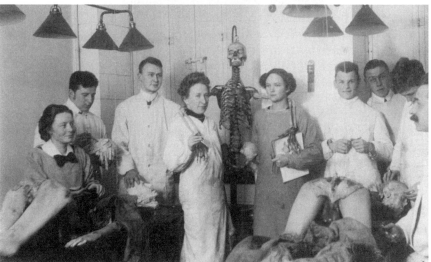

Figures 6 and 7. Photographs from the dissection room, Academy of Surgery, Copenhagen, ca. 1910 (photographer unknown). Medical Museion, University of Copenhagen.

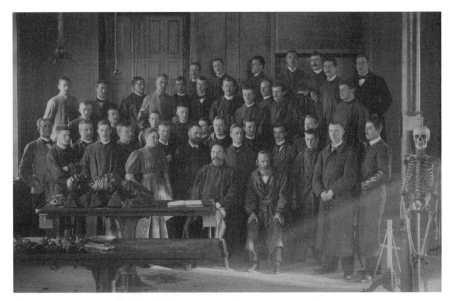

Figure 8. Professor Edvard Clason surrounded by students in the dissection room, Department of Anatomy, Uppsala University (undated, photographer unknown). Maps and Prints, Uppsala University Library.

Laughter and dark humor functioned as defenses against the fear of death and were part of the grotesqueries of carnival culture. Yet medicine had to defend itself and its aristocratic discourse against such grotesqueries. It was thus necessary that the education of medical students include training in handling corpses in a way that concealed the grotesque.[87]

Few photographs survive of anatomical milieus in Sweden around the turn of the twentieth century. Among these photos, I have found none that show joking and grotesqueries. Most of these photographs are of an altogether different nature: they show medical students in large or small groups, standing at dissection tables on which corpses lie.[88] They resemble other group or class photos, but the often central placement of the corpses makes them special, more like pictures of hunting groups with their freshly killed trophies. These pictures also have associations with the group portraits from earlier centuries that show scientists with their objects of study.[89] If anatomy course dissections are considered an initiation into medical science and training in a special way of regarding dead bodies, then such pictures are also symbolic diplomas.

In an undated photograph from the Department of Anatomy at Uppsala University, Professor Clason (seated, with beard) is surrounded by a large group of students (see figure 8). One member of the group is a woman. Most of the students are wearing dark protective lab coats, and a few also wear sleeve protectors. On the left side of the picture are two dissection tables. On the foremost table lie objects that could be the legs of the torso on the other table. These human remains and the skeleton placed farthest to the right in the photo, almost as though it were another student, provide the attributes necessary to identify the scene as the anatomy department. As a rhetorical gesture, a book lies open on one of the tables; the combination of practical dissection experience and textual studies would give the students anatomical knowledge.

Gender and Power in Anatomical Work

All the anatomists and pathologists mentioned to this point were male. This is symptomatic, since the milieus examined in this study were populated almost exclusively by men. Men were teachers, professors, authors of textbooks, lecturers, students, and custodians. Medical science's single-gendered, homosocial environments maintained male collegiality and team spirit. In the internal histories of the various medical departments, tone-setting teachers are depicted as father figures, persons of genius, and charismatic leaders.[90]

The majority of the dissected bodies were male, and most of the illustrations in textbooks depicted male bodies. In medicine, as in many other disciplines, the male was the "normal case," and the female was the exception. In the textbooks, female bodies were presented primarily in their role as producers of children. Medical students encountered females mainly in the anatomy and pathology of the sexual organs and the uterus. As Professor Edvard Clason is said to have stated, "Woman is nothing more than a case for her uterus."[91]

All the women anatomist Erik Müller and his colleagues at the Karolinska Institute encountered in their daily work were subordinate to them. They were either sick, and thus in a position of dependence, or dead, and subjected to the male physicians' cutting instruments and scientific gaze. Some were nurses and thus professionally subordinate. Eventually, female medical students began to be admitted, but for a long time they were few in number, and they had to adapt to the prevailing culture at existing medical schools (there were no all-female schools). For many years, they found themselves outside the social circles and scientific clubs that had been established by men for men, who did not want women among their numbers. The first female physician, Karolina Widerström, graduated in 1888, and in 1938 the Karolinska Institute—and the country of Sweden—welcomed its first female endowed professor, Nanna Svartz.[92]

The history of the role of women at the Karolinska Institute and other medical institutions has yet to be written. These women are barely mentioned

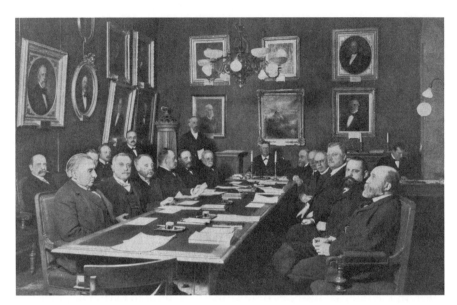

Figure 9. "The professors of the Karolinska Medico-Surgical Institute gathered in their meeting room." A homosocial milieu. Photograph by Axel Malmström. From *Hvar 8:e Dag* (December 18, 1910): 182. Duplication: Kungl. biblioteket - National Library of Sweden.

in the official histories of these institutions—it is the men's history that was recorded. In his history of the Department of Pathology at the Karolinska Institute (see figure 9), Carl Sundberg mentions a female teaching assistant and three female drawing assistants.[93] Israel Holmgren mentions in passing Hilda Magnusson, a laboratory cleaning lady at the Karolinska Institute's medical clinic who became "a skilled preparer of specimens, who cured, bedded, cut and colored brain sections."[94]

The professional women who first gained entrance into scientific milieus were assistants and artists. Only men held positions of authority, and the assisting women worked to make possible the men's research and teaching activities. While male assistants were often medical students who needed practical training or an income for a certain period and then advanced to more prestigious positions, women were often limited to a lifetime as assistants. During the nineteenth century, the need for laboratory examinations for health care and medical research increased. The number of assistants in the institutions grew, and the division of labor became more obvious, as Swedish historian Bodil Persson has shown in her book on the history of laboratory assistants. According to Persson, this division of labor developed "into a separation of work into technical processing and scientific analysis.

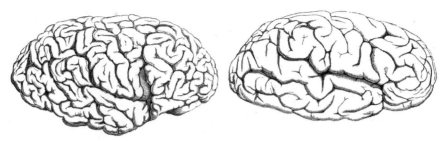

Figure 10. "Motion increases the number of muscle fibers, 'thinking' increases the number of convolutions of the brain." On the left, the brain of the mathematician and astronomer Carl Friedrich Gauss; on the right, that of a manual laborer. Woodcut and quote from Carl Reclam, *Menniskokroppen, dess byggnad och lif: Populära föredrag* (Stockholm: Ad Bonnier, 1884), 68. Duplication: Kungl. biblioteket - National Library of Sweden.

Specialization had begun, with the handiwork going to the women, and the science to the men."[95]

Women were not only deemed socially subordinate to men; they were also considered biologically subordinate. On the whole, they were viewed as inferior human beings, weaker, more unstable, and less refined than men—in fact, inferior to men in all areas except caregiving, raising children, and managing the home.[96]

Yet in the hierarchy established by scientists in the late nineteenth and early twentieth centuries, not only women were classified in the lower levels. Anatomical methods were utilized in comparing the bodies and brains of different races and ethnic groups. Brains were weighed, measured, and examined in regard to structural complexity. Scientists believed a connection could be seen between greater structural complexity and a more highly developed capacity for reason. Highest in the hierarchy of brains were, not surprisingly, those of white European males: in particular, learned men, gifted artists, the anatomists themselves, and their friends. The brains of women and workers were believed to be smaller and lighter and to have fewer convolutions (see figure 10). Even farther down the scale were non-European ethnic groups. The lowest of all was the "Hottentot" woman, whose brain was judged as having the same level of intelligence as a European idiot. It was felt that these results had been reached through scientific methods, based on systematic anatomical comparisons.[97] This is just one example of how science was racialized.

Anatomical instruction also bore the stamp of gender differences, as can be seen in two Danish photographs from around 1910. The photos show classes in anatomy for nursing students at the Danish National Hospital and for surgical students at the Danish Academy of Surgery, respectively. The

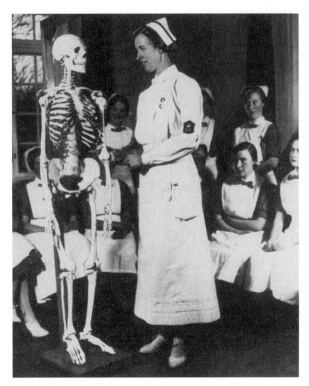

Figure 11. Nursing students receiving instruction in anatomy, National Hospital, Copenhagen, 1910. Medical Museion, University of Copenhagen. Photographer unknown.

differences are striking. The nursing students, in neat white caps and aprons, sit or stand in a half-circle around the teacher (see figure 11). The female teacher in full nursing uniform, with white stockings and shoes with decorative bows, stands facing a skeleton. She and the skeleton are about equal in size and look as though they are talking to one another. Besides the comical dimension of this obviously arranged photo of a class lecture, the situation glows with propriety, purity, control, and freshly washed linen. Even the skeleton looks neat and well-groomed.

The second picture has a more documentary flavor (see figure 12). A group of men wearing lab coats stand in a room with tiled walls, surrounding a corpse they are in the process of dissecting. One of the men seems to be the person in charge, the teacher. He looks straight into the camera. His clothes are different from those of the others: his starched collar is higher, and a necktie and jacket can be seen under the dark lab clothing. With his

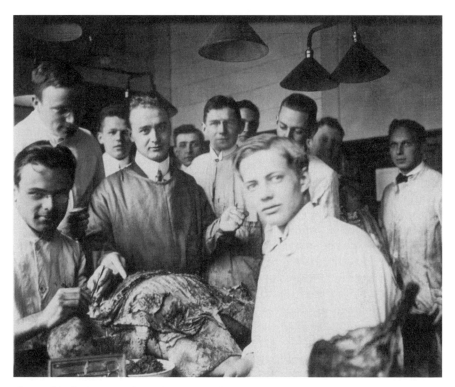

Figure 12. Surgery students dissecting a body under the direction of Otto Agaard, Danish Academy of Surgery, ca. 1910. Medical Museion, University of Copenhagen. Photographer unknown.

right hand he points to the opened cadaver, while his left hand holds a cigarette. (It was common to smoke during dissections, to make it easier to withstand the smell of corpses in an era of nonexistent ventilation.)[98] Beside the teacher sits a man with a scalpel in one hand and a pair of tweezers in the other. Some instruments in a case can be glimpsed in the lower left edge of the photograph, next to a bowl containing organic material. Some of the men in the picture are blurred because they are in motion, further strengthening the sense that the photograph was taken in the midst of an ongoing exercise.

In contrast to the still portrait of the nursing students, this one is not well organized—the men are in motion; they are wearing soiled, wrinkled lab coats; they are smoking and engaged in the work. Further, their cadaver is not pleasant to see. If anatomy instruction for female nursing students was a pure and primarily theoretical activity, for male surgical students it was practical, hands-on, corporeal, and dirty.

This chapter has examined the attitude of medical science toward dead bodies and the conflicts to which this attitude gave rise, as well as how legislation was formulated with regard to shifting ideas about who had the power of decision over a body. The results support the earlier findings of other researchers in this area, who have pointed out that in the modern era, authority over death shifted from the religious to the medical sphere.[99] Yet power over the body, living as well as dead, is charged with issues of class, race, and gender. Medical science's strong position around the turn of the twentieth century included the privilege of ranking the different segments of humanity. These rankings were made by white Western men who had built up medicine's position in society, and they did so with the help of the anatomical sciences.

The tension between the beneficial and grotesque aspects of the cut-up dead body was a problem for physicians and for medical discourse. For those outside the discipline of medicine, both the instrumentalist and the jokingly cynical attitudes toward death were perceived as offensive. The view of the body as useful for the advancement of science and medicine is a modern phenomenon: it began with Vesalius and his followers in early modern society, culminated in modernity (in the late nineteenth and early twentieth centuries), and began to fade in late modern society—as did doctors' position of power. In the deepest sense, perhaps the aversion to anatomical dissections expresses a resistance to the medical attitude that corpses can be made useful. When anatomists made death a servant of humanity, they created a symbolism that clashed with other roles death had played in cultural history. Through dissections, deceased persons were transformed into dead bodies—into objects. In the hands of doctors, death and the dead were made anonymous and profane. It is not surprising that this situation gave rise to protests.

It is also not surprising that at the end of the nineteenth century the general public found it difficult to allow their relatives' dead bodies to undergo clinical or forensic autopsies. This procedure was not part of the ritual forms of handling corpses—the passage rites that were necessary for life to return to normal. The doctors who wanted to conduct autopsies had completely different views. For them, cutting into dead bodies was a matter of course within the realm of medical activity. It was an everyday practice, as indicated by the quotation introducing this chapter, in which cutting into a brain is compared to slicing a loaf of bread. Eventually, however, the autopsy was normalized, and by the end of the twentieth century it was no longer perceived as a disruption of the ritual order. The autopsy became a modern rite of passage; identification of the cause of death is now considered vital to create order and meaning.[100]

Dissections and autopsies were vital for the production of knowledge in anatomy and pathology departments of Western medical schools. But the doctors and students did more than cut into dead bodies; they also devoted much time and effort to preparing and preserving body parts. Bones, organs, and tissues needed sophisticated treatments to become accessible for research and study. Chapter 3 compares professional medical museum collections and displays to those of popular wax museums, where deviance and death were put on display.

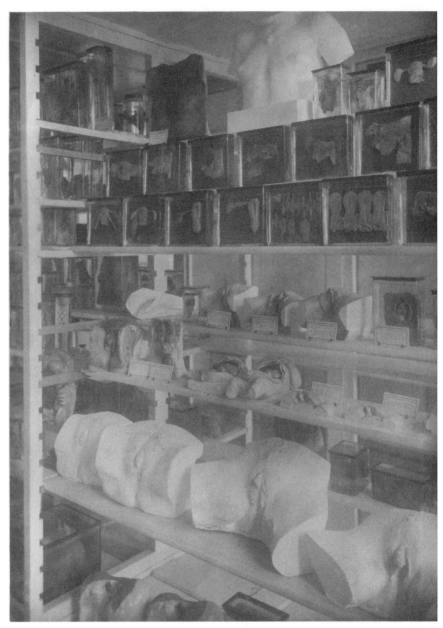

Figure 13. Female and intersexed ("hermaphrodite") genitals on display in an anatomical museum. From Gaston Backman's 1925 photo album, Riga, Latvia. Maps
and Prints, Uppsala University Library.

Chapter Three

Death on Display

Around 1900, the Karolinska Institute's facilities at Kungsholmen in Stock-holm housed several museum halls. Glass cases, drawers, and shelves were crowded with systematically organized pieces of bone, skeletons of animals and humans, body parts dried or preserved in liquid, and plaster casts of body parts, normal or diseased. There were also entire human bodies and organs modeled in wax.[1]

Similar artefacts were on view at Lütze's Plastic Wax Museum on the island of Kungliga Djurgården in Stockholm. The displays there showed exotic eth-nic groups, scantily clad women, courageous heroes on voyages of discov-ery, and infamous criminals—all in wax, with real human hair and authentic clothing. There was also an anatomical section, with models of the develop-ment of the fetus in the uterus, sexual organs afflicted with horrible diseases, a bladder stone operation in cross-section, and more. In addition, objects that had once been alive were displayed: a mummified child, the stomach of an alcoholic, and the dried skin and penis of an African "native."[2]

The Karolinska museum was closed to the public and was professional in nature. Its visitors were students, researchers, and their assistants. The Plastic Wax Museum was a commercial, popular museum. Despite their dif-ferent purposes, the items exhibited in the two museums were surprisingly similar. How could this be? This chapter examines how dead bodies were used as objects of display in various settings and how death came to be part of the spectacular, modern visual culture that flourished around the turn of the twentieth century.[3]

Anatomy: A Visual Culture

On the evening of April 24, 1894, the Swedish Society of Medicine (Svenska Läkaresällskapet) convened in its offices on Jacobsgatan in Stockholm. As on every Tuesday, a meeting was followed by an informal gathering, with food and drink.[4] The main event that evening was a lecture by Gustaf Retzius on how organs could be preserved by curing them in formalin. The technique was new, and Retzius had tested it with success. The method was especially well suited to brains (unless they were from fetuses and thus too small). Retzius had brought several cured human brains with him, which he showed to his colleagues. He also exhibited cured calf, pig, and dog eyes, as well as the heart and liver from a cat.

The Swedish Society of Medicine had been established in 1808 with the goal of forming an exclusive medical academy. The society became, however, a Stockholm-centered doctors' association that pursued both scientific and social activities. Its facilities housed a meeting hall, a library, and a social room. Membership grew rapidly around the turn of the century, from 361 members in 1881 to 884 by 1908.[5] At the Tuesday meetings, members presented lectures and discussed issues involving medicine and hygiene. Meetings were especially lively when the topic was a current issue, such as the recurring cholera epidemics. The meetings were private, but minutes were kept and published as *Förhandlingar vid Svenska Läkaresällskapets sammankomster* (*Proceedings of the Swedish Society of Medicine*). Beginning in 1839, the society also published the monthly journal *Hygiea: Medicinsk och farmaceutisk månadsskrift,* in which particularly interesting lectures from the meetings were published, and the print series *Svenska Läkaresällskapets Handlingar* (*Transactions of the Swedish Society of Medicine*).[6] The leading physicians were also influential at the Karolinska Institute, including Anders Retzius and, later, his son Gustaf, as well as the latter's work partner for many years, Axel Key. All three men were also researchers and teachers in the anatomical sciences.

Lectures that dealt specifically with methods of preparing specimens were relatively rare at the Swedish Society of Medicine. More frequently, doctors would present tumors or organs that exhibited pathological changes. Sometimes, they showed living patients with interesting diseases. Another long-standing tradition was to provide detailed reports from the autopsies of famous persons, especially royalty.[7] Case descriptions were regularly presented and included reports on the progression of a disease, treatment, and autopsy results, as well as occasional specimens. Depending upon the nature of the condition, the specimens might be individual organs, systems of organs, or particular tissues. A typical example was the case of scurvy in combination with cancer on which Axel Key reported in April 1874 discussed in chapter 2. The specimen was a piece of spinal cord tissue that Dr. Key described in detail and compared with drawings of other specimens of spinal tissue.[8]

Until his death in 1901, Key was the Karolinska Institute's leading pathologist. During his years as chair of the Swedish Society of Medicine, he dominated the group's activities in the field of pathology. *Svenska Läkaresällskapets historia,* the history of the association published in 1908, describes some of the areas in which he had special interest—primarily "the study of tumors; a significant number of tumors from all portions of the body, mostly malignant, are demonstrated" but also "blockages of the intestines" and similar phenomena.[9]

Monsters, or malformed fetuses, were also presented. For example, the 1876 *Svenska Läkaresällskapets förhandlingar* described how Gustaf von Düben showed an alcohol-preserved fetus with two deformations: hydrocephalus ("water baby" syndrome) and extra fingers and toes.[10] When Frithiof Lennmalm summarized the scientific portions of the society's meetings for 1835–1858, he noted: "As usual since the earliest days of the Society's meetings, a large number of malformed fetuses were shown, as well as congenital deviations of all sorts."[11] In the summaries from later periods, malformed fetuses are no longer mentioned. However, deformities continued to be presented in *Svenska Läkaresällskapets förhandlingar*, although perhaps to a lesser extent than during the first half of the 1800s. Research on malformations continued to be pursued within the areas of teratology and embryology.[12]

The preservation of pathological body parts was an important element in physicians' activities. The presentation of rare cases or new discoveries was, then as now, a matter of prestige among doctors. The advancement of medical science and the education of physicians were typically cited as key parts of the mission of professional medicine. The Karolinska Institute's vast collections of both normal and pathological specimens had been built up through the doctors' collecting and preparation of material.[13] Doctors from around the country also sent interesting specimens to the experts at the Karolinska. When Retzius demonstrated the new method of preserving organs in formalin to the society in 1894, it was thus of interest to many of those present.

Chemical curing makes it easier to handle an organ and thus makes it more accessible for examination. Unless an organ is studied immediately when the body is opened, it must be cured or preserved. It is important that the preservatives do not cause significant changes to the organ.[14] In his lecture, Retzius related how difficult it could be to cure a brain, for example, and how important it was to find a method suited to the purpose.[15]

Brains may be cured to retain their natural shape and volume, if their natural membranes are left intact, and they are hung by a thread tied to the *art. basilarus* in a 0.5% solution of formalin, which must be changed after 24 hours. The coloring agents of the blood are drawn out by the preservative liquid, and the gray brain matter takes on a somewhat darker gray color. After 7–10 days, the curing process should be concluded. By this time, the brain matter, if it was reasonably fresh when the process was undertaken (1–1½ days after death) will have taken on an elastic, "pillow-like" consistency; the convolutions may be easily folded open. . . . This curing method is in all cases well suited for the study of the convolutions of the brain and other coarser morphological details, not least in consideration of educational requirements. The cost is extremely low. . . . The advantages of this method will quickly be seen. As is known, in curing by spirits, the brain shrinks markedly and becomes quite hard, while in curing by formalin, shape and volume are maintained, and the consistency becomes soft and elastic, so that *gyri* and *sulci* are with much greater success made accessible for closer inspection. Judging from the experiments performed thus far, the formalin method is also well suited to the preservation of many other organs, especially in cases of macroscopic examinations and museum preparations.[16]

Practice(s), Techniques, and Visual Representations

An anatomist's working matter consists of dead body parts. The practical ways of handling this material are central to anatomical knowledge production as well as to the everyday experience of working with anatomy. This is true of all anatomical disciplines, even if their focus and methods differ. Anatomical instruction also has special, historically changing requirements. Dissection was a central part of medical education around the turn of the twentieth century, crucial for the performance of a modern medical professional identity, in Sweden as elsewhere in the Western world.[17] Dissection exercises on embalmed corpses were combined with other methods of instruction, such as the study of textbooks and preparations. Lectures played an important role, and the visual representations of objects of anatomy were key pedagogical aids. A photo from the Department of Anatomy at Uppsala University shows an array of visual materials for a lecture on the anatomy of the brain (see figure 14). A large model of the brain stands in the center. Grouped around it are schematic drawings, posters, and diagrams, along with a drawing on the blackboard.

Toward the end of the nineteenth century, research interests within the anatomical sciences were focused on the small structures: tissues and cells. Research in normal anatomy was conducted primarily within the field of histology. For the histologist, a microscope was prerequisite, and the material to be studied had to be prepared in special ways. Usually, a tiny portion of cured, colored tissue was sealed in a protective layer of paraffin and then cut into millimeter-thin slices using a special device known as a microtome. Emil Holmgren, professor of histology at the Karolinska Institute, published a textbook, *Lärobok i histologi,* in 1920. In the first chapter, forty-five pages were devoted to "microtechnique"—methods for preserving, dividing, coloring, injecting, mounting, and modeling.[18] In addition to illustrations of microscopic cell preparations and a microscope with various objective lenses, Holmgren also included a picture of a microtome, along with a description of how it worked (see figure 15).

The quality of preparations could vary, of course, and it was of great importance to master and develop techniques that would produce preparations that revealed what they were supposed to reveal and allowed one to see what needed to be seen. Next, the anatomist had to interpret the specimen and communicate the findings to others. All of this was dependent upon the

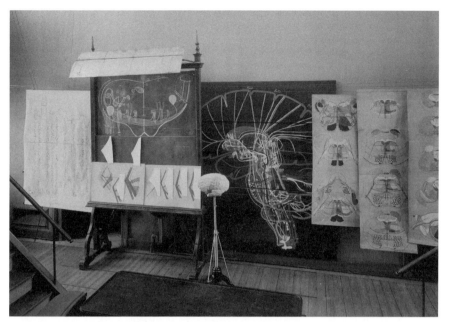

Figure 14. Visual materials for a lecture on the anatomy of the brain, Department of Anatomy, Uppsala University, probably from the late 1880s (photographer unknown). Maps and Prints, Uppsala University Library.

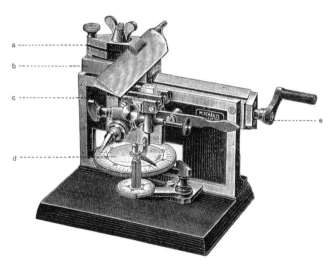

Figure 15. A microtome, a device for slicing specimens. Illustration from Professor Emil Holmgren's textbook, *Lärobok i histologi* (Stockholm: Norstedt, 1920), 15. Duplication: Kungl. biblioteket - National Library of Sweden.

quality of the researcher's preparation, technique, and skill, as demonstrated by an 1873 article in *Nordiskt medicinskt arkiv*, "Om lymfvägarna i magsäckens slemhinna" ("On the Lymph Vessels in the Mucous Lining of the Stomach"), by Christian Lovén.[19] Lovén had successfully examined the occurrence of lymphatic ducts in the stomach linings of humans, sheep, calves, rabbits, dogs, and cats using a special technique described in his article. For mucous membranes to be studied under a microscope, they first had to be dissected, preserved, and sliced in appropriately sized pieces. In addition, they had to be colored by injecting liquid into the lymphatic ducts, which would otherwise be invisible. In the article, Lovén described various injection methods, as well as the best types of needle, cannula, and coloring agent. Aesthetic values were important: Lovén preferred a beautiful blue shade of iron vitriol (Prussian blue), and for red he used red ferric cyanide in water.[20]

The scientific results of Lovén's experiments were thus dependent upon a technique used to make them visible. The development of this technique was in turn dependent upon the formulation of the scientific problem. Analysis of the material was made using the researcher's eyesight and a visual instrument, the microscope. In addition, communication of the results of the study (the scientific article) contained graphic elements (illustrations), which were at least as important as the textual ones. N. O. Björkman, the Karolinska Institute's artist, produced drawings of the preparations selected for inclusion in the article, which were then transferred to lithographic plates to be published as pictures (see figure 16).[21]

A memorial article on the recently deceased Viennese anatomist Josef Hyrtl, written by Gustaf Retzius in the 1894 edition of *Hygiea*, further demonstrates the importance to anatomists of the ability to prepare specimens. Hyrtl had given Retzius a valuable "collection of masterfully prepared, rare animal skeletons," which had been added to the Karolinska Institute's anatomy museum and which provided "a beautiful testimony to Hyrtl's mastery of anatomical techniques." The gift also included a collection of microscopic injection preparations, "which in their day elicited general admiration, and had been awarded prizes at the world's expositions."[22] Clearly, Retzius felt Hyrtl's scientific discoveries were a result of his skill with his instruments:

> The dissection knife and chisel were his primary instruments, and *with the hypodermic needle, he made excellent discoveries* in the macroscopic anatomy of the vessels of the body. . . . His preparations of the muscles, vessels and nerves were the most complete of their sort, and have provided the basis for a very large number of essays and monographs which he has published, primarily in the comparative and descriptive areas of the study of human anatomy.[23]

This summation makes clear that the anatomical sciences are visual disciplines that deal with differences and similarities in the structure and color

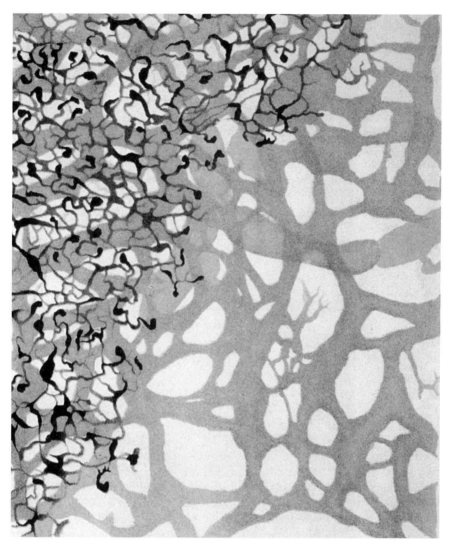

Figure 16. A portion of human stomach lining; lithography made after a drawing by N. O. Björkman. The original has mild, transparent colors that range from a light, yellowish green-gray to evening blue. From Christian Lovén, "Om lymfvägarna i magsäckens slemhinna," in *Nordiskt medicinskt arkiv*, vol. 5, no. 26 (Stockholm, 1873). Duplication: Kungl. biblioteket - National Library of Sweden.

of large or small parts of normal and pathological (human and animal) bodies. The presentations of preparations and pedagogical dissections for students, as well as autopsies and scientific research on the structure of tissues, are thus determined by visual impulses.[24] It is vital and necessary to make things visible. What cannot be seen cannot with certainty be said to exist. The consequence of this fact is that techniques for making things visible and (re)presenting them are of decisive importance.

The quality of visual anatomical representations is dependent upon a series of advanced practices that result in pictures strongly controlled by the conventions of their genre. A high degree of prerequisite knowledge is required for the viewer to take advantage of the pictures, which are not just simple reproductions of reality. Lovén's images of mucous membranes are constructed and mediated in several steps and are meaningless without the contextual text.[25]

Part of the construction of an anatomical image involves the seldom-discussed fact that the specimen is a (portion of a) dead body, while the knowledge the anatomist seeks and wants to convey deals with living bodies.[26] Drained blood vessels are depicted as full of blood, and the colors shown are not those of a corpse but those of a living body. Even the colors follow established conventions—in reality, veins and arteries are not bright blue and red, yet in anatomical illustrations they have been shown in these colors for hundreds of years.

The Anatomist's Gaze

Whether in scientific articles or textbooks, anatomical and pathological writing contains numerous references to the visual, sight, and the gaze. Edvard Clason's speech at the dedication of the new dissection hall at Uppsala in 1884 is typical of the ways turn-of-the-century anatomists discussed their work (and resonates of many anatomical texts since Vesalius). This section analyzes Clason's use of expressions associated with gaze and images.[27]

According to Clason, the goal of anatomy instruction is that the student obtain "as complete a knowledge as possible of the human body," a knowledge not fully developed until one can "see through the folds of the body." This is to be achieved through one's "own observations, i.e., one's own work and own observation with an avid, searching gaze."[28] The individual who does not do this risks becoming as ridiculous as someone who has taken his or her travel memories from a guidebook only, although "[k]nowledge gathered beforehand from a textbook can, of course, provide an occasional ray of knowing, especially in the eyes of the unknowing." Used properly, however, the textbook can be used advantageously, in part to verify one's own observations and in part to make the student more observant of things that might easily go unnoticed. One's own preparations should be compared to the textbook "as new views open themselves, and as new individual observations are made."[29]

Observations made during the actual handling and study of anatomical parts generate pictures in the memory that, according to Clason, last longer than the memory of the pictures in study prints. Students are encouraged to imprint the memory of each preparation in their minds, "as if it were a picture of the dearest object, which you might never again be allowed to regard."[30] According to Clason, illustrations should be used with caution. He cites the French anatomist Philibert Constant Sappey, who in his anatomy textbook wrote that unhappy is the student who exchanges nature itself for a pale copy because he or she sees nothing and is unwilling to see anything.[31] Memory is likened to an album filled with the images one has retained: "since in the end, a hasty summary of all the anatomical pictures in this album is necessary, do not seek your brush strokes and colors only in the somewhat faded pictures of the textbook."[32] The clearest memory pictures are obtained from well-made preparations, which should be clean and neat; even though not everyone is capable of producing beautiful and attractive preparations, they should at least be well-crafted.

Different pictures may compete with one another. The schematic image may be of assistance in this regard, but it can also be dangerous "by forcing the memory picture" out of the mind. The best method, according to Clason, is to personally draw pictures of preparations from memory and then verify their accuracy. In this way, an individual may learn to see the shortcomings in his or her own observations. If drawing is difficult, create pictures in the memory instead, training the "inner capacity for the production of pictures" and "paint[ing] in one's imagination."[33] Clason feels it is especially injurious to depend upon textbook knowledge in regard to the skeleton. Here, the student ought rather to study preparations, as well as the student's own living body and the bodies of others, on which the student can practice by feeling the skeleton through the flesh. One must dare to rely upon one's own experiences: "Why not see with one's own eyes before putting on the glasses offered by others, to see in a dependent way from their viewpoint and with their capacity to break light, which may not correspond to one's own."[34] Practice dissections are intended not only to imprint anatomical knowledge but also to develop the capacity for observation, which is of central importance to the work of the physician.[35]

The visual culture of anatomy thus consists not only of visual aids such as pictures and anatomical preparations. The gaze, vision, and capacity for observation are central to the work and necessary for both gathering and developing knowledge. This is true of anatomy both as an educational subject and a field of research. The production of new anatomical knowledge requires that the anatomist sees something new and is able to represent it for others to see and judge. That which cannot be seen does not exist.

The anatomist's work is intended to make the body visible and legible; the language used to describe this work contains numerous words linked to seeing and pictures. Aesthetic evaluations abound—a preparation or even the color of a dissected kidney can be described as beautiful. Descriptions are often colorful and pictorial; they require the translation of visual impressions into verbal language to call forth an understandable vision for the reader. Anatomists are thus trained in visual skill on several levels above and beyond the capacity to make observations at the dissection table. They should be able to interpret different types of illustrations and preparations; they must be able to produce good pictures and preparations; visual impressions must be preserved as pictures in the memory, as a knowledge bank for future comparisons; they must be able to translate visually obtained knowledge into words, and the language must be clear so it can be understood by other anatomists. The capacity to "paint in words" is perhaps even more important for pathologists than for anatomists. They must be able to show how the diseased body differs from a healthy one and how one kind of diseased tissue differs from another, using color and texture as important keys.

The Anatomy Museum

During the nineteenth and early twentieth centuries, each department of anatomy, pathology, and physiology maintained its own collection of preparations of various types—a departmental museum. This was true of the Karolinska Institute and the departments at Lund and Uppsala universities, as well as of medical facilities throughout the Western world. The museums were filled with body parts from floor to ceiling. The anatomical collections in Uppsala are recorded in a photograph that shows numerous display cases containing neatly organized preparations (see figure 17). In the foreground are large dry preparations of lungs, and above them are labeled jars containing small wet specimens (organs preserved in liquid).

These museums functioned as reference collections for clinics and researchers. At the same time, the museum served as a repository of educational and instructional materials for medical students, a place where they could train their capacity to see through the use of specimens prepared by their teachers and predecessors. The museums also served as memorials to highly skilled anatomists, and the collections were admired for the beauty of their preparations.[36]

The Karolinska Institute's anatomy museum was superb, containing most of the common types of preparations. After the Department of Anatomy acquired new facilities in 1886, the museum was housed in nine rooms.[37] There were several rooms of skeletons and skeleton parts (the osteological collection) from common and rare animals of all sizes and humans of all

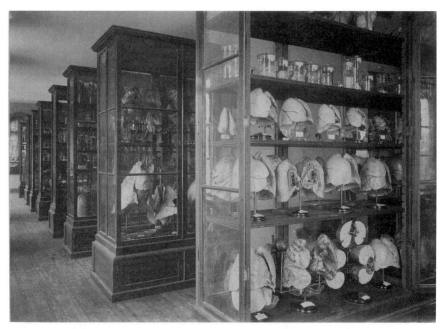

Figure 17. Anatomical Museum, Department of Anatomy, Uppsala University. Photograph probably taken in the late 1880s (photographer unknown). Maps and Prints, Uppsala University Library.

ages from various parts of the world. Anthropologist Hjalmar Stolpe donated skulls of Incas and Polynesians, "as well as the complete skeleton of a Japanese"; Gustaf Retzius, Christian Lovén, and E. Nordenson donated sixty Finnish skulls; fifty Sami skeletons excavated at Varangerfjord in Norway were purchased for 1,500 crowns, and the museum also received the skulls collected by members of A. E. Nordenskiöld's Vega expedition.[38]

The skull collection was crucial for research in physical anthropology, which focused on identifying distinguishing anatomical traits of the human races. The practice of racial science was widespread in Europe and North America from the late eighteenth century onward, and the anatomists at the Karolinska Institute contributed enthusiastically to this world-encompassing practice. Physical anthropology was a special interest for both Retzius the elder and the younger.[39] Anders Retzius developed an influential system for classifying the races according to their cranial shape, which remained in use long after it was introduced in the 1840s. The basis of this system was the classification of groups into longer (*dolicocephalic*) and broader (*brachycephalic*) skulls, in combination with prominent (*prognathous*) or flat (*orthognathous*) lower jaws. Skulls classified into races according to this method were drawn by students at the Royal Academy of Fine Arts, as can be seen from a drawing by Erik Lindberg as late as 1894.

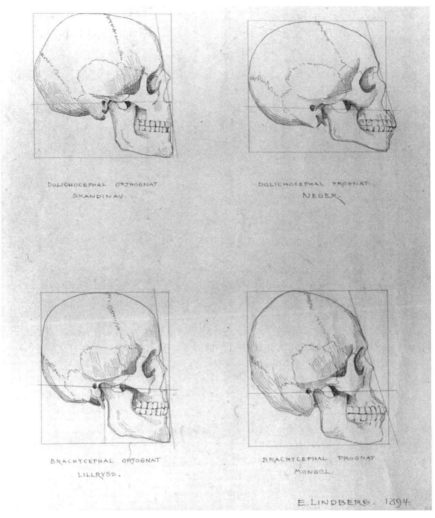

Figure 18. Skulls drawn according to Anders Retzius's anthropometric system. Erik Lindberg, *Four Skulls,* 1894. Photograph by Göran Persson. Royal Swedish Academy of Arts, Stockholm.

The anatomy museums also contained wax models of entire human bodies and organs, plaster casts, and both normal and diseased organs preserved by various methods such as drying and formalin. The collections were continually expanded through donations and preparations of interesting material. Special areas were set aside for specimens prepared by each method. In addition to the museums' display areas, storage rooms held preparations used in classroom instruction.[40]

In 1910, when Erik Müller, professor of anatomy, wrote a history of his department in the *Karolinska mediko-kirurgiska institutets historia,* he described the museum's excellent collections and the efforts made to improve and maintain them. He also reflected on how the department's needs for materials and collections had changed over the years as the research had taken on new directions:

> During the period of time which has passed since Anders Retzius founded the Karolinska Institute's anatomy museum in the 1830s, the meaning of an anatomy museum has to a certain degree changed. During a time when the development and completion of systematic and topographic anatomy came about with the aid of increasingly minute preparations or the discovery of new methods of preservation and injection, the organization of display collections was a natural result of the scientific study. . . . In our present time, when the emphasis in scientific anatomy is upon comparative anatomy, descriptive and experimental embryology and the statistics of variation, *laboratory work* has taken the place of museum work. In accordance herewith, efforts during the most recent period have been directed not so much toward the procurement of objects for display, as toward the collecting of valuable zoological and embryological material. In this respect, the Museum is in the possession of quite a respectable [collection of] material.[41]

Although the museum's "display collections" had become less important by the early 1900s, dead body parts were still collected and preserved for research and educational purposes, although in ever-smaller formats.

Anatomy and Art

Anatomy was a subject not only for doctors-to-be but also for artists. European artists and anatomists had been collaborating since the Renaissance. While artists were afforded the opportunity to study the structure of the human body by drawing dissected corpses and anatomical preparations, anatomists also benefited from the help of artists in producing visual material for research and instruction. In academic programs for the education of artists, students received a thorough immersion in the structures of the human body. Drawing practice used not only living models and classical sculptures but also anatomical representations and preparations. The schools' educational material included skeletons and bones of humans and animals as well as écorchés (sculptures of skinned human bodies revealing the muscles).[42] A painted écorché of a male body from the eighteenth century is still kept in the cellar of the College of Fine Arts in Stockholm, although it has lost its head and arms. This écorché has been drawn innumerable times, and it was used as a model for drawing practice at least until the end of the nineteenth century. A drawing by Erik Lindberg of the torso of the écorché serves as an illustration of this special type of visual representation, which was based on sculptures or casts of dead human bodies (see figure 19).

Art students also gained practical experience with dissection. During Anders Retzius's time as professor of anatomy at the Royal Academy of Fine Arts, classes using corpse materials were held at the Karolinska Institute's facilities.[43] Carl Curman, who held the same post from 1869 to 1902, had been a student at the academy (see figure 20).[44] During his time there, the academy moved to a new building with a well-lit corner room for dissections, a storage room for anatomical preparations, and a special elevator for bringing corpses up from the street level. These facilities were used from 1897 until around 1920. Anatomical dissection gradually lost its importance in art instruction, but as late as the 1950s the academy's anatomy teachers brought their students to the Karolinska Institute, where at least once during their anatomy course they would study preparations and attend a dissection.[45]

For artists, knowledge of anatomy was not a goal in itself but rather a means for learning how to portray the human body. What role did dissections play for art students? Why would they want to touch body parts, smell the nauseous odor of the anatomy hall, and see the "gnawed-off human remains" on the dissection tables (as the famous Swedish artist Carl Larsson expressed it)?[46] Would prints, models, and skeletons have been sufficient? If anatomy exercises could train medical students to maintain a clinical distance, what was the goal of the art students' encounters with dead bodies? Was it that nothing human should be foreign to them or that they were to learn to see through their models? The use of dissection exercises in art education was a holdover from an era when science and art were more closely bound together than was the case in the early 1900s. Symbolically, however, medicine and art were linked through the practice of anatomy until well into the modern period: artists were initiated into the fleshly secrets of medicine, and doctors learned to see and to draw what they had seen.

The Body as Spectacle

Anatomical science was not the only cultural arena for exploring the human body's curious forms. Anatomical preparations, models, and prints, as well as people with all sorts of physical deviations, were also exhibited in a completely different cultural sphere: public entertainment. Theses popular spectacles had much in common with anatomical museums and shared a pre-history in the collections of remarkable objects in cabinets of curiosity (so-called Wunderkammer).[47] For example, in the eighteenth century the natural history collection at the royal palace at Drottningholm displayed a giant's hand in plaster, a wax model of the dwarf Bébé, and portrait busts of two dead young princes.[48]

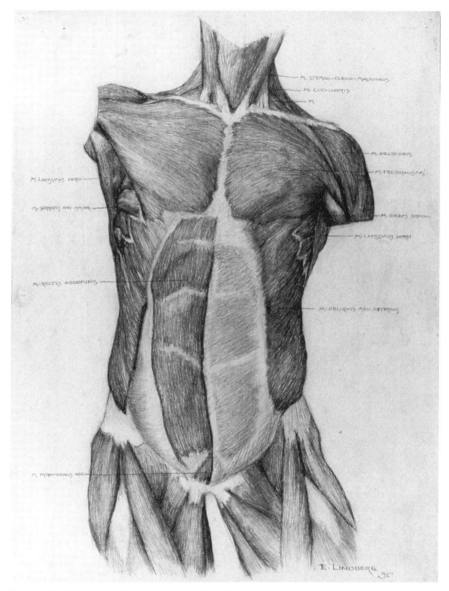

Figure 19. The model for this anatomical drawing was an écorché, a painted plaster sculpture of a flayed body. Erik Lindberg, *Torso*, 1895. Photograph by Göran Persson. Royal Swedish Academy of Arts, Stockholm.

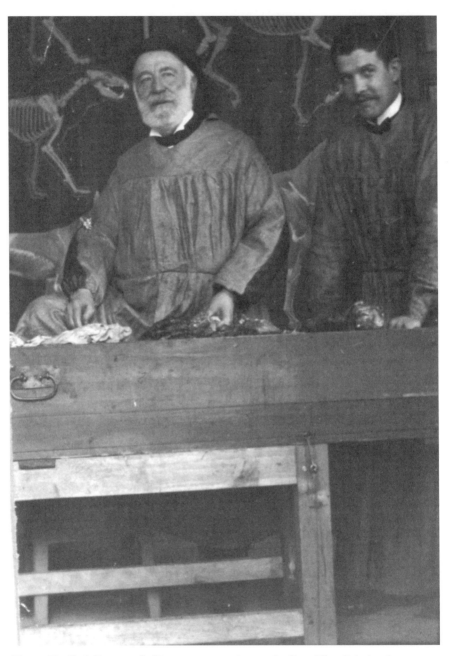

Figure 20. Carl Curman (left), anatomy teacher at the Royal Swedish Academy
of Arts, and his assistant, 1899 (original photographer unknown). Photograph by
Göran Persson. Royal Swedish Academy of Arts, Stockholm.

Wax has been used as a modeling material and in various aesthetic contexts since antiquity. Models for the casting of bronze statues, medals, and coins were made out of wax.[49] It was also used to cast extremely realistic portraits, such as the medieval and early-modern funeral sculptures of kings and queens preserved at Westminster Abbey in London.[50] Italy has a several-hundred-year-old tradition of creating dioramas depicting biblical motifs, for which the figures were often made out of wax, and ex-votos in the form of wax limbs were on display in churches and chapels.[51]

During the eighteenth century, it became increasingly common for medical schools to commission wax models (casts and sculptures of normal and pathological anatomy). These models served instructional purposes, allowing students to study the structures of the human body in detail. Veterinarians, zoologists, and botanists also had study aids created in wax. The most famous eighteenth-century wax sculptures are from Italy, many of which can still be seen in Bologna and Florence.[52]

Scientific and medical collections were systematized and diversified during the nineteenth century, in connection with the increasing specialization of scientific disciplines. The curiosity cabinet's tradition of eliciting a sense of wonder was continued and developed in the sphere of public entertainment. Oddly shaped people and animals, living or dead, were exhibited in the salons of the bourgeoisie and in tents at fairs and markets. Scientific exhibitions were distinguished from the more public and commercial ones primarily through the method of organizing and exhibiting them. The objects could be more or less the same, and the boundaries between science and spectacle were fluid.[53] For example, the Hunterian Museum, now housed at the Royal College of Surgeons in London, had one of the most distinguished scientific displays in the early nineteenth century. It contained the skeleton of the "Irish Giant," Charles Byrne (8 feet, 2 inches), next to the skeleton of the "Sicilian Dwarf," Caroline Crachami (20 inches); exotic peoples, either in portraits or stuffed; and rows of normally or abnormally developed fetuses in glass jars.[54] By the end of the century, this eclectic practice of displaying anatomical and pathological curiosities was still common in the entertainment world, while medical museums were reorganized according to new scientific systems.

Wax Museums around 1900

The turn of the twentieth century was the heyday for wax museums. The Royal Library in Stockholm has a collection of brochures, catalogs, and posters from wax museums. Its oldest catalog was printed in 1849 and the most recent in 1945, but most are from the years 1880–1920. At least two of the wax museums that existed in Sweden have been preserved, one in Jönköping and one belonging to theater owner Per Simon Edström of Nacka. The latter is Lütze's Plastic Wax Museum, which was shown at Gröna Lund in Stockholm until 1920. Many other wax museums varied in size, quality, and level of ambition. Some went on tour to other countries.[55] Some focused on current events and famous persons of the time; others were religious in nature, and still others were simple sideshow spectacles.

The more inclusive wax museums featured both current events and titillating sensations. A number of wax museums went by the name "panoptikon." This term stems from the Greek words for "everything" and "see"—it was thus the place where one could see everything. Wax museums typically claimed to offer visitors almost everything that might pique their interest. Models of exotic people and curious artifacts from cultural and natural history were common elements, but the exhibitions also often included an anatomy section. To be able to see the interior of the human body portrayed in the extremely illusionistic medium of wax was, in other words, a public pleasure and an attraction at that time. Wax figures were also exhibited in other contexts. At the 1897 Stockholm Exposition, dioramas with wax figures were shown at the Biblical Gallery and the Sports Pavilion.[56] Artur Hazelius used this technique as early as the 1870s in his Scandinavian ethnographic collection on Drottninggatan in Stockholm. One of the dioramas there featured a wax version of a painting by Amalia Lindegren that was widely known through popular prints, showing a heart-wrenching scene of a weeping mother at her child's deathbed.[57]

Sweden's best-known wax museum was the Swedish Panopticon (Svenska Panoptikon). It filled four floors of a building adjoining Kungsträdgården Park in Stockholm in the years 1889–1924. On display there, probably inspired by the Musée Grévin in Paris, were wax sculptures set in lavishly produced scenes of famous events. The figures were sculpted by artists working with live models. The studio also accepted works on commission.[58] Numerous extraordinary scenes could be viewed, ranging from the royal family having coffee in the palace to Swedish explorer Sven Hedin in the Mongolian desert. Oddly, a portrayal of anatomist Axel Key was an object of display, sitting in the Lagerlunden café at the old Stockholm Opera House with some of his friends.[59] Death and terror were featured elements in the Swedish Panopticon (as well as in the touring wax museums), represented in the death scenes and death masks of several famous persons; down in the cellar, murderers and grave robbers stood in chilling dioramas (see figure 21).[60]

Anatomy, Hygiene, and Pornography

Touring wax museums advertised their attractions through posters. "Hartvick's Anatomical Panopticon and Wax Museum" came to the town of

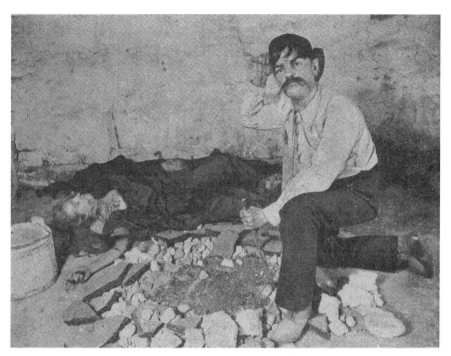

Figure 21. Diorama with the British-Australian serial killer Frederick Bailey Deeming and one of his victims, in the Swedish Panopticon's "Cellar of Terror" (photographer unknown). From *Vägvisare genom Svenska Panoptikon* (Stockholm, 1895), 39. Duplication: Kungl. biblioteket - National Library of Sweden, Ephemera Collection.

Vetlanda in March 1915 (see figure 22).[61] Its poster is rather simple and has no pictures. The headlines announce most of the attractions common to the wax museum. In addition to themes dealing explicitly with representations of human anatomy, Hartvick's Panopticon also lured visitors with "Famous Persons. Crowned Heads. Torture. Preparations from Nature, etc." The exhibit tried to stay current: "Several Leading Men from the World War" were included. Behind these non-anatomical topics was a peculiar corporeality: the entire concept of wax museums and their justification for existence lay in the concrete portrayal of human life in a bodily form. The purpose of showing famous persons was the same then as it is today at Madame Tussaud's: to give the visitor the experience of being in the same room as famous personalities, who (are supposed to) look as though they are truly present in bodily form.[62]

The name of this museum, Hartvick's Anatomical Panopticon and Wax Museum, emphasizes its anatomical content, which is specified in summary form on the poster. A portion of the exhibition is claimed to be a "scientific, anatomical special exhibit," in which the human body is shown in wax figures

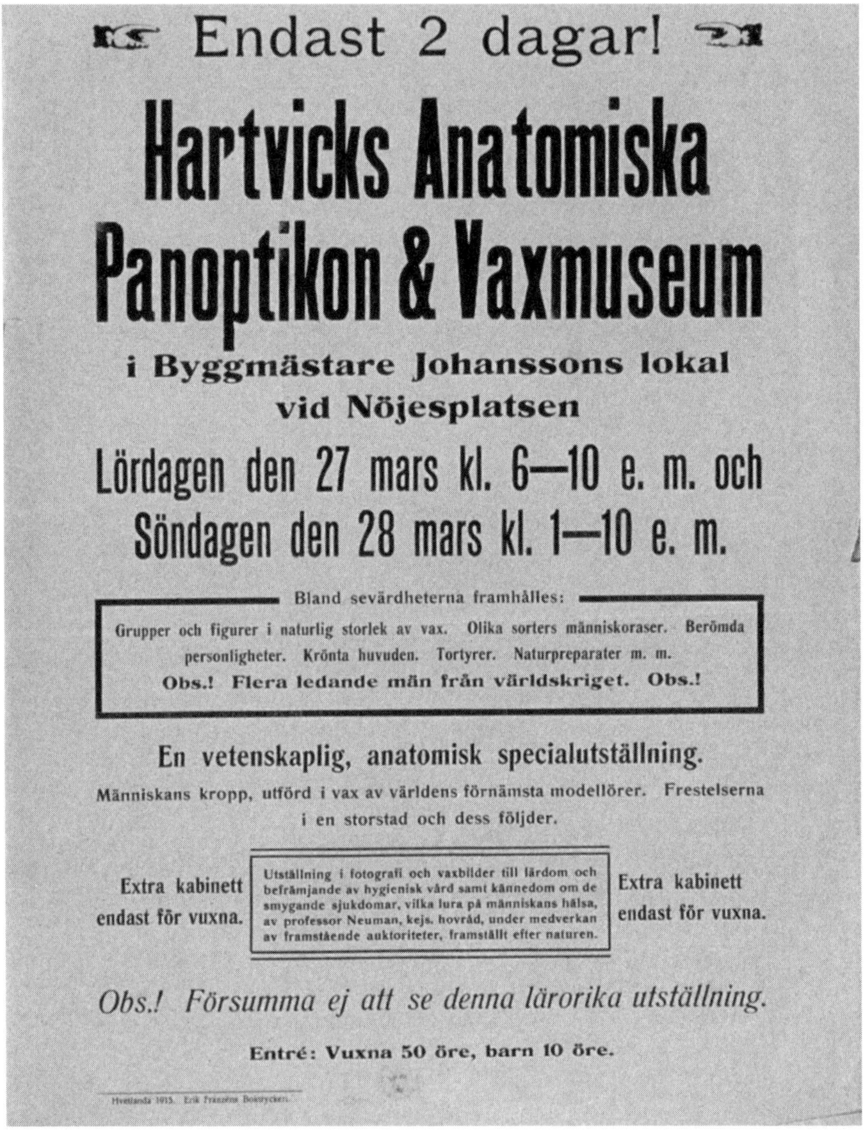

Figure 22. Poster advertising Hartvick's Anatomical Panopticon and Wax Museum in Vetlanda, with "a special scientific anatomical exhibition" as well as celebrities, torture scenes, "natural specimens," and more, 1915. Poster Collection, Duplication: Kungl. biblioteket - National Library of Sweden.

made by "the world's foremost model makers." The opportunity to see representations of the human body is emphasized, as is the high quality of the models. The words "scientific," "anatomical," and "special" rhetorically give the exhibition an air of legitimacy and respectability. At the same time, these words advertised an open display of intimate body parts.

The poster heading "Extra Display for Adults Only" implies that the contents of the exhibition could be morally challenging. The line is displayed on both sides of a rectangle that contains this message:

> An exhibit of photography and wax models for instruction in and the promotion of hygienic care, and for knowledge of the insidious diseases which prey upon the health, executed by Professor Neuman, court advisor to the Kaiser, under consultation with prominent authorities, modeled from life.

This proclamation signaled that the exhibit would likely show representations of sexually transmitted diseases, inner organs destroyed by alcoholism, women's bodies deformed by corsets, and other features that might upset children. It was meant to attract adults to this display of risqué subjects while simultaneously balancing acceptable morality. Tension between the seedy and the moralistic is also implied by the heading "The Temptations of the Big City and Their Consequences."

The marketing rhetoric of wax museums made use of known and unknown authorities to legitimize the exhibitions. Here, advisor to the German kaiser, a Dr. Neuman, and unnamed "prominent authorities" are mentioned. How well Neuman was known in Sweden was of little importance—what mattered was his title. The names of scientists and prominent professors were often used to assert the credibility of exhibits. Some did lend their names, but others were probably mentioned without the person's permission. The Swedish physiologist and public health educator Anton Nyström endorsed Castan's Museum of Anatomy, among others. Nyström's guarantee of quality is quoted in the exhibit catalog:

> The undersigned has viewed Castan's Museum of Anatomy, and hereby certifies that it contains a rich collection of well-executed and true-to-life depictions, as well as preparations from nature, which are interesting and educational for persons seeking knowledge, especially those who through popular scientific lectures may have achieved some insight into anatomy and human health.
>
> Stockholm, Dec. 4, 1908.
> Anton Nyström, Doctor of Medicine.[63]

Health, hygiene, and knowledge are words of honor here, helping to give the impression that wax museums such as Castan's were idealistic establishments for the promotion of popular medicine. Public educational museums of hygiene did exist. For example, Anna Hierta-Retzius (married to Gustaf

Retzius) donated a museum of hygiene that was housed in the old facilities of the Karolinska Institute's anatomy department. The museum was open to the public and was said to have been well visited, although what it contained is unclear.[64]

In Paris, a wax museum from the second half of the nineteenth century still exists, the Athaeneum, Muséum anatomique et Ethnologique. It was created by a doctor, Pierre Spitzner, who added new sculptures to an older collection of anatomical waxes. Spitzner's express purpose for his exhibition was to promote improved health among the populace under his motto "Science—Art—Progrés."[65] For his museum, Spitzner assembled a hygienic section, consisting mainly of waxes depicting male and female body parts, mostly genitals and faces afflicted by syphilis. The purpose of this section was to teach members of the military to avoid contracting syphilis.[66]

Musée Spitzner, as the collection is known today, is one example of a wax museum that was established with the intent of educating people. Not all commercial wax museums with anatomical displays sought to improve public health and contribute to improved public knowledge, however. Some, in fact, had little or no legitimacy. The goal of public education, which was compatible with the health and hygiene discourse of the day, was just one theme among many for the wax museums. The same objects that were designed to enlighten people could also provoke completely different thoughts and feelings. Certainly, wax museums had less noble goals—for example, to make money by attracting as many visitors as possible through spectacular and sensational displays. Spitzner's exhibition, like those of other wax museums, made the most of the modern interest in science while still appealing to a popular taste for the grotesque.[67]

Anatomical and hygiene-related displays were problematic. Tension existed between scientific education and pornographic titillation. The wax museums' claims of scientific value should therefore be viewed with a critical eye. These claims should instead be seen as strategies for forging associations with science and public education, which were positive phenomena at the time. Wax museums thus tried to win legitimacy with the middle classes and legal authorities while also displaying sexually explicit material. The fact that a wax figure was scientifically correct did not preclude it from depicting a curvy woman clad in diaphanous clothing, reclining indolently on satin cushions.[68]

From its inception in 1882, the Parisian wax museum Musée Grévin consciously avoided anatomical displays to keep from being associated with the allegedly pornographic wax museums.[69] The contemporaneous Swedish Panopticon in Stockholm also excluded anatomical specimens and models. Like the Musée Grévin, it claimed to be a better, more respectable entertainment establishment, with refined displays suitable for the modern middle class.[70]

Dead and Abnormal Bodies as Attractions

Julia Pastrana was an attraction, a performer not only during her lifetime but after her death as well. Pastrana, known as "the Ape-Woman from Mexico" or "the Baboon Woman," toured the world performing a song and dance routine and was described by male observers as polite and engaging, despite her unfeminine face. Her entire body was covered with thick, dark hair, and her nose, ears, and jaw were unusually large. These traits were inherited; in recent literature her condition has been classified as "congenital hypertrichosis with gingival hyperplasy."[71] The story of Pastrana's life is fascinating, and a worthy analysis could be made of her position in the cultural hierarchies of her day, based on perspectives of gender and race. Here, I discuss Pastrana as a frequent figure in the world of wax museums. She was modeled in wax, and she was even displayed after her death, stuffed and mounted, together with her embalmed, hairy newborn child (see figure 23). She died in Moscow in 1860 at age twenty-six while on tour with her American husband, her impresario in life and in death.[72]

On a Swedish poster from the 1860s, Pastrana is touted as one of the attractions in a "LARGE ANATOMICAL MUSEUM." Pastrana's name and description are given central placement and a large amount of space on the poster.[73] The poster emphasizes that this is the genuine Pastrana, not a copy. The text uses words such as "her," "dancer," and "mother" while simultaneously referring to her as "this unusual creature" and "this rare example." The embalming of Pastrana's body is described as skillfully done, something in itself worth seeing: "She died in childbirth three years ago, and was, along with her child, so masterfully embalmed that it has gained the admiration of all of the men of Science in Paris and London."

It is as though Pastrana's status is unclear; it falls somewhere between human being and something else, perhaps animal or thing. This lack of clarity was utilized in marketing her performances during her life: she was sometimes described as a missing link between ape and human. These claims transformed Pastrana's body into an object that did not have to be treated with the same respect as other dead human bodies and that could be viewed by all with a clear conscience. They also made the display of her body marketable. At the same time, the poster text tells about Pastrana's life, thus evoking an image of a recognizable human being. Based on her appearance, which was said to unite "ape and human physiognomy," she was placed in a zone that stirred the imagination of those captivated by Darwin's still relatively new theory of evolution.[74]

The ontological uncertainty in the statements about Pastrana is disturbing today and was presumably so in the time when they were written. Her public image was constructed as a borderline case, an attraction in and of itself in a culture that devoted great effort to defining its boundaries and

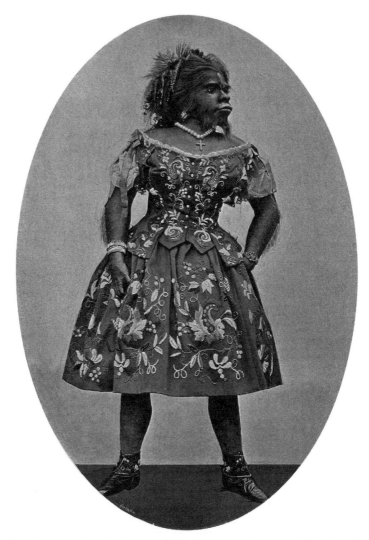

Figure 23. Photograph of the deceased Julia Pastrana, who was exhibited to the public in Sweden as late as 1973. Courtesy of the Wellcome Library, London.

organizing its categories.[75] Pastrana's physiology challenged the delineations between male and female, human and animal, with her hairy body and heavy features combined with an ample bosom, delicate feet, graceful dance moves, and a lovely singing voice.

The poster text about Pastrana's embalmed body displayed many of the marketing themes used by other wax museums about other objects: it was described as *authentic* and *sensational;* a *female body* that could be viewed for a fee, without moral considerations; her ethnic background was *exotic;* she was a *famous person* who was also *dead;* she was exhibited as a *physical oddity;* she was perhaps regarded with *fear.*

Death, Visuality, and the Body

The use of wax models, as I have shown, linked the cultures of medicine and entertainment. Another link was the use of dead body parts for display. Death was constantly present in the exhibits, in part in objects made from human body materials and in part in exhibit topics and themes: murder and murderers, grave robbing, the death beds of famous persons, death masks, executions. The different display domains were especially united in their interest in murderers and other executed criminals: casts of criminals' heads and hands were included in both professional and popular medical museums. This section describes the relationship of scientific anatomical visual culture to commercial spectacles.

Exhibitions of the abnormal in wax museums were based on the notion of the healthy white male as the norm. The ideals of normal life were constructed through the display of the abnormal, the diseased, and the criminal—wax museums' greatest attractions.[76] Through its organizational practices, medical science participated in the same cultural project—a project that used dead bodies as instruments. The opening, separating into parts, and conserving of dead bodies may be regarded as a prerequisite for both modern anatomical science and popular exhibitions and thus for the construction of categories such as normality, gender, sexuality, and race.[77]

A deviant human body could be valuable both in life and in death, for both the wax museums and medical science.[78] Historians Robert Bogdan and Rosemary Garland Thomson have shown that many of the persons exhibited as "freaks" in the United States were also used as research objects by pathologists and teratologists, both during life and after death.[79] The attraction of the unusual for both science and the entertainment world was a result of the way it challenged the defined boundaries of nature and culture. Julia Pastrana occupied a liminal position, intermediate between cultural categories constructed as opposite one another, or dual: man/woman, normal/abnormal, nature/culture, human/animal.[80] The embalmed object, the corpse on display, can be placed into yet another liminal position: a state between life and death. This liminality of the corpse was challenging in and of itself.

During the nineteenth century, deviant bodies came to be defined less as "oddities" or freaks of nature and more as a pathological deviation. The freak show had close ties to medical discourse, but after the turn of the twentieth century the two went their separate ways. Medicine's cultural position grew stronger and was imbued with an aura of authority and prestige, while the common freak shows declined and were labeled vulgar and immoral. Thomson connects the decline of freak shows to the fact that medical science had turned those with deviant bodies into medical objects. This "medicalization" transformed them into disabled persons. Well into the middle of the twentieth century, doctors visited freak shows to find study objects, and the showmen exploited science to give their exhibits believability and authenticity.[81] Both the medical world and the world of spectacle objectified unusual or deviant bodies and used them for their own ends.[82]

Thomson's analysis of the relationship between freak shows and medicine can be transferred directly to the relationship between wax museums and medical science. Dead bodies were exploited just as much as deviant ones, often because they, too, were deviant. Wax museums also gradually lost popularity and began to disappear during the interwar years. This was in part connected to the process of medicalization, although it was not the only reason.

Wax museums were part of the visual culture of the nineteenth century, which included other popular entertainment such as panoramas, dioramas, picture magazines, stereoscopic photographs, lantern slides, and, eventually, moving pictures.[83] What made wax museums special was the medium: wax offered the possibility of producing hyper-realistic representations of the human body. The material itself was extremely well suited to portrayals of various aspects of human life and death. Using oil paints, a skilled wax sculptor could make the surface look like living skin; with the addition of real hair, the illusion became almost total. The wax museum offered unique opportunities to see remarkable human phenomena in life and death, up close. During the second half of the nineteenth century, wax museums presented titillating spectacles of bodies and body parts, as well as tableaux of current events. But in the early 1900s they began to receive stiff competition from films, which seemed more "modern."[84] The anatomical wax museum, like other visual amusements introduced in the 1800s, was replaced by new forms of entertainment. The need for anatomical and pathological study material in education and research diminished simultaneously. Anatomical collections thus lost their audience and their justification for existence at roughly the same time.

To understand the similarities and differences between popular anatomical wax museums and professional medical museums, consider the changing and variable meanings of the term "museum." The two museum types used the same name and displayed the same sorts of objects. But their cultural context differed, and so did their relationship with the public; thus the meanings of the objects they exhibited diverged.[85] When popular wax museums used the name "museum" and sought authority through certificates from famous academicians, they showed their dependency on science and the exhibition culture of the times while simultaneously taking a lower position within the hierarchy of exhibitions.[86] An object that had been displayed at a world exposition could lend authority and legitimacy to the display objects in both types of museums.[87] When touring "museums" showed their deformed fetuses in formalin and their stuffed bodies, they offered the general public the same sorts of objects that were displayed in elite medical schools and were manufactured using the same techniques and aesthetics. Yet the objects took on different meanings in different settings. The relationship between artefacts and the public is complex. The persons who decide which objects to display and how to display them have only partial control over the reactions of viewers, who respond intellectually, emotionally, and imaginatively.[88] Swedish medical historian Karin Johannisson has described how even when presented in a scientific context, old display items can send chills down a viewer's spine: "Of all the objects in the Museum of Natural History in Gothenburg, I was as a child irresistibly drawn to a special artefact pressed into a glass jar: the Siamese twins, who with closed eyes floated in their eternity of yellowed, slightly muddy spirits."[89]

Scientific exhibits cannot be regarded as purely rational, constructed along entirely practical and scientific lines. Wax museums, for their part, were neither merely spectacular and pornographic nor purely scientific and disciplined. Rather than two separate phenomena, medical and commercial exhibition practices were part of a larger culture of display. They exhibited unity with a broad spectrum of venues, forms of expression, and audiences. Medical museum collections were most numerous and largest during the late nineteenth and early twentieth centuries, the same period in which the popular wax museums enjoyed their golden age. These two forms of cultural expression, which at first glance seem so different, shared a number of organizational methods and practices and were parts of one visual culture, with the body, death, and deviance at its center.[90]

The culture of exhibiting death and dead body parts flourished around 1900 but did not survive in modernity (although it has made a comeback in recent years, with the popular traveling shows of "plastinated" corpses, such as "Bodyworlds" and "Bodies"). The custom of viewing the deceased before a funeral is another form of death display that has virtually disappeared in modern Sweden. Chapter 4 explores what happened when professional funeral directors took over the task of preparing the dead body for the funeral from persons closer to the deceased, a process that removed death from most people's sight.

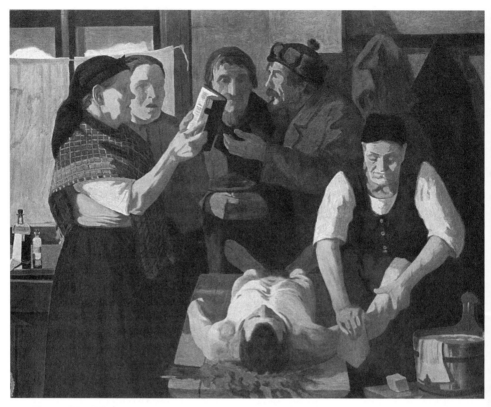

Figure 24. Oil painting by Juho Rissanen (1908) with an unusual motif: the washing of a corpse. The painting is owned by the Museum of Art in Turku, Finland. From the Photo Archives, Nationalmuseum, Stockholm.

Chapter Four

Preparing the Dead Body

According to ethnologist Yvonne Verdier, in some small French villages a "help-wife" was relied upon at death as well as birth. The help-wife helped the newborn into the world if no professional help was available or acted as an assistant to a midwife or doctor. She also washed and clothed the village's dead.[1] When Verdier did her study in the 1970s, the eighty-five-year-old help-wife Marcelline told her how things used to be done. Marcelline had learned from her mother, who had been a help-wife before her. The tradition went as far back as at least the early twentieth century, and Marcelline had been able to follow the changes introduced into death rituals. Even in the 1970s, funeral homes were not yet established in this rural area.

When someone died, the help-wife managed the associated tasks. The body had to be washed and its hair nicely arranged; if the deceased was male, it had to be shaved. The help-wife then dressed the body in fine clothes and laid it between clean sheets. She closed the eyes and mouth, hid the face under a handkerchief, and folded the hands over the stomach, which was decorated with a rosary and a twig of boxwood. The prepared body lay in a room for three days, with someone keeping constant watch over it. In earlier times, neighbors had helped, offering to sit with the deceased for several hours each night. In the period following World War II the tradition of watching over the corpse disappeared. Yet in the 1970s the body still had to be cleaned and groomed, even though the number of people who would see the body had been reduced to one: the help-wife herself.[2]

The help-wife's tasks at both birth and death were similar in a very concrete way: she washed and clothed bodies; she cleaned rooms and put them in order; she arranged beds and the areas around them with clean towels and sheets, which were also changed and washed. The items she used for both jobs were the same—a washbasin, water, and linen—simple, everyday things that took on a ritual function. The help-wife's washing of the newborn and the dead carried meanings above and beyond the hygienic.[3]

According to Verdier, the dead body was understood to be dangerous, yet despite (or because of) this it had to be cared for. It was important that the person who performed these tasks was unafraid and "invulnerable."[4] The help-wife's tasks rendered the corpse harmless: washing the body purified it; hanging a cloth over the mirror in the room prevented it from retaining the image of the deceased; keeping watch over the deceased protected those associated with the dead person in life. "The job of the help-wife is to domesticate, humanize, socialize," Verdier wrote.[5] The villagers saw women as the givers of both life and death, which explained why it was always women who cared for the newborn and the dead. Death was understood to be a result of the Fall, which Eve had caused.[6]

This chapter deals with the ways modernization transformed caring for dead bodies in Sweden. Preparing bodies for burial was largely a task for local women in nineteenth-century rural Swedish culture. In modernity, it became a service provided by professionals for payment.

In her fieldwork, Verdier became intimately acquainted with Marcelline's life and was able to describe her functions and position in her village. No similar study exists of a Swedish "help-wife." In Sweden, the modernization of rural areas occurred much earlier than it did in the region of France Verdier studied, and the traditional patterns of living she found in the 1970s would no longer have existed in Sweden. Swedish ethnologists of the early twentieth century studied peasant customs and traditions, but not in the way Verdier did and not with the same theoretical framework.[7] They did, however, leave behind a body of material that makes it possible to study how the dead were cared for in rural Swedish agricultural society before the patterns of modern society had become established there.

The picture of traditional ways of dealing with dead bodies that emerges from the archives of the Nordic Museum in Stockholm is similar to the methods described by Verdier. Yet beginning in the final decades of the nineteenth century, the handling of dead bodies underwent a gradual but thorough process of change that was completed by the 1940s. The practice of paying a funeral director to manage the details surrounding death and burial spread from the upper levels of society to the lower classes and from city to countryside. The archival material consists of reports and excerpts recorded by museum staff and colleagues on ethnographic field trips throughout Sweden, covering the period from the mid-1800s to the mid-1900s.[8]

I have also used replies to the Nordic Museum's questionnaires (and the preparatory work that preceded them). For example, in 1958 the museum sent a questionnaire to funeral directors throughout Sweden, with questions specifically about "the Traditions of Undertakers." In addition, I have used publications of the Swedish Association of Funeral Directors (Svenska Begravningsentreprenörers förbund). This material provides a window into the practices of handling dead bodies and how the work of undertakers came to replace traditional practices.

Washing, Enshrouding, and Clothing the Dead

In Sweden, as in France, it was usually women who washed and enshrouded the dead. "An older woman called 'Mother Lisa' was the one who clothed dead bodies," wrote a correspondent for the Nordic Museum in 1962:

She was also the one who was relied upon when a baby was born. She made everything so neat and pretty, in times of both sorrow and joy. She was there and showed us children the deceased. We were to lay our hand upon the brow of the deceased, so that no one would be afraid afterward.[9]

According to ethnologist Ulrika Wolf-Knuts, the washing of corpses was strictly a women's task among the Finland Swedes she has studied.[10] As will be seen in the section on the washing of corpses that follows, the Swedish material reveals that men also washed dead bodies. But reports of men clothing bodies are rare.

The picture that emerges from the archives is complex—customs and traditions varied from place to place and time to time. Furthermore, in certain localities people seem to have been less particular about death customs, while in other areas people held tightly to the way things were "to be done." The reported variations depended upon the informants, as well as on how the recording ethnographers perceived and understood the situations. These variations are perhaps the most interesting part of the reports—it cannot be unequivocally stated that things were done one way or the other in "the old days." Nevertheless, the stories documented in the archives share some common characteristics: the dead had to be taken care of, and there were rituals regarding how this was to be done; the bodies were washed, clothed, and laid in coffins; the corpse was viewed by those saying farewell to the deceased. The ways these acts were performed varied, though, as did the manner in which the coffin was transported to the cemetery, how and where the committal ceremony was conducted, and related customs.

One conclusion that can be reached is that the dead body was perceived as significant. The practices were charged with meaning, but what was most important was that they were carried out. To gain an overview of the degree to which these practices changed during Sweden's modernization, this chapter first examines the ways the dead were handled in rural Sweden during the second half of the nineteenth century.

Washing and Shaving the Deceased

In rural Sweden the bodies of the dead were sometimes (although rarely) washed by men, especially if the deceased was a man. In her 1937 study, folklorist Louise Hagberg mentions that in Gårdby on the island of Öland, this job was assumed by the local tailor or church deacon.[11] He also neatly arranged the hair of the deceased and shaved the beard stubble. An old man from the province of Blekinge in the early 1900s remembered a childhood encounter with death and the washing of a corpse:

> I remember that my grandfather lay in the bedroom in our house. His corpse was placed on the lid of a bench which stood on two chairs, with a sheet draped over him. First, they sent for a man who shaved corpses. He shaved and washed the dead man, so that he was nice and clean before his final earthly journey. I remember so well how this man stood in our cottage and shaved my grandfather, who had died at our house, and then washed him with a cloth, and dried him off with a towel. I was 7 years old, and I thought that it looked odd. I was quite shy about this, and my reaction was a little bit of fear toward the dead man.[12]

The Nordic Museum questionnaires reveal a division of labor between men and women: women more commonly washed and dressed corpses of both sexes; men shaved and trimmed the hair of male corpses. Men might also lay the body in the coffin, since this task required physical strength.[13]

In 1927, an eighty-year-old working-class woman from Öland told Hagberg that it required a special person to "wash up" corpses, since not everyone would "consider doing it."[14] In certain places, it was important that the person who washed the body was not a relative. If a newborn baby died, the task might fall to the child's godparents.[15] An undertaker from the town of Värnamo related that when he had been an apprentice in the 1920s, an old woman of the parish washed the corpses. He maintained that it might have been many years since the person had washed, so it was necessary to use "strong soap and a brush" to get the body clean.[16]

The reports concerning customs surrounding death contain many details about how to deal with objects that had been in contact with the corpse and items that had been removed from it, such as hair, beard, and nail trimmings. Such items were to be rendered harmless in more or less specific ways, often in connection with the washing of the body. In particular, many stories describe what was to be done with the wash water. It was often left in a vessel under the bier and thrown out after the funeral procession.[17]

In the reports, explanations of the motivations for washing the corpse are not uniform (this is a basic problem: the ethnographers asked about customs and traditions but not about the respondents' ideas regarding them). Some respondents believed the deceased had to be clean when they stood before the Lord or when they entered the realm of the dead, which was not always the same thing. There are hints of belief in a continued existence in which the dead live on and continue in their trades and social relationships. In a 1926 report, Brynhild Wilén recorded a statement by a farmer in the province of Värmland in which he reflects on how the ways of washing corpses had changed:

> When they wash bodies now, they don't do [it] like they did in the old days; back then, they used to say that they should be clean when they came to heaven, so they washed the entire body of the deceased. Now they only wash the parts that can be seen.[18]

Clothing the Deceased

The dead also had to be clothed before they were laid in the coffin. Regarding the decoration of corpses and coffins in the second half of the nineteenth and the early twentieth centuries, recall that many people came to view the deceased and to say farewell (a custom that has virtually disappeared in Sweden). The corpse was shown both when it had been prepared and was awaiting burial and before the funeral procession, when the funeral guests gathered for the final journey to the cemetery.[19] The coffin was open. The lid was put in place just before the procession began. The corpse had to look good in its coffin for this final showing.[20]

Many reports describe the enshrouding of the deceased. Although the Swedish term *svepning* implies "enshrouding," this rarely meant that the dead were wrapped in fabric. According to many informants, the corpses of married adults were clothed in the shirts or blouses they had worn on their wedding day.[21] Certain informants indicated that special full-length linens were sewn during a person's lifetime and saved for enshrouding his or her corpse.[22] White socks were often put on the feet of the deceased, and mittens or gloves were sometimes put on their hands.[23] A woman could also be dressed as a bride, either with a linen slip, veil, and bridal crown or in a complete bridal costume, including shoes and gloves (see figure 25).[24] Even young unmarried women and girls were often dressed in a veil and a bridal crown.[25] In 1950, on behalf of the Nordic Museum, Karin Hanses interviewed elderly women in Leksand parish in the province of Dalarna, all of whom had many years' experience clothing deceased persons. Their descriptions show that people took pains to create a fine appearance, using what was available: bridegrooms' shirts, fine scarves, different types of hats for married and unmarried women, and ribbons and roses made of glossy paper.[26]

Some of the informants carefully described the clothing of the dead in detail and considered the customs important. Others ascribed less significance to the clothes. For example, one undertaker related that around the turn of the twentieth century, before commercially made burial clothes could be purchased, the dead were buried in whatever underclothes were available in the home.[27] (This could also be a covert way of claiming conditions were worse in the days before professional undertaking.)

Burial clothes varied in appearance and changed over time. In 1928, a ninety-three-year-old woman from Stöllet in the province of Värmland, who in her younger years had sewed many burial shrouds, reported that the most common burial attire was a simple shroud that covered the deceased up to the chin. Sometimes, the deceased's hands were laid over the shroud. There were seldom any decorations other than perhaps a few flowers, which became more common later as more cultivated flowers became available. When a child's body was prepared, it had to be especially pretty, and the

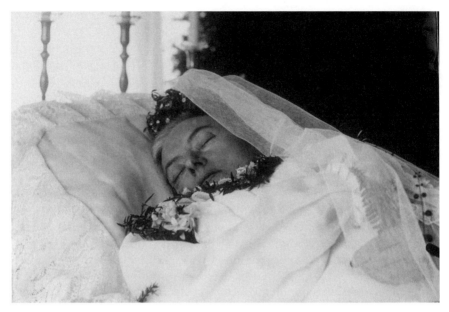

Figure 25. Deceased woman dressed as a bride. Photograph by Otto Johansson of Furusund, Sweden (undated, ca. 1910–20). Stockholm City Museum.

coffin was decorated with artificial roses, silk ribbons, and tassels.[28] Other reports verify that extra care was given to dressing dead children.

Children, both girls and boys, could be "shrouded in a cloud" (*svepas i sky*), which meant that tulle or some other sheer fabric was laid over the body or stretched over the coffin.[29] Most often, white and black cloth was used for the clothing of corpses, with colored accents in the form of green twigs or artificial flowers made of glossy paper. Sometimes, however, the colors of traditional wedding costumes or children's clothing were bright. They are especially vibrant and imaginative in a funeral scene Hagberg described from the province of Södermanland in the 1880s: a dead girl lay in her coffin, clothed in a pink dress. Around her, blue fabric was arranged like a sky, decorated with fluffy clouds of white fabric.[30]

Sexuality

The archival material rarely mentions sexuality. It is thus particularly interesting when such references do appear. From the province of Skåne, there are several reports of "the covering cloth" or "covering rag" (*skyllelapp, skyllepalt*). This was a piece of cloth about the size of a handkerchief that was placed over the lower abdomen of the deceased, under the other grave clothes, to conceal the genitals. A woman from Skåne born in 1866 said it was very important that the person who dressed the corpse not forget the "covering cloth," for the blessedness of the deceased depended upon it.[31] In another report, a farm wife remembered that when her father died in 1912, her aunts checked to be sure the covering cloth was in place underneath the grave clothes.[32] Hagberg claims that this custom derives from a belief in physical resurrection and from representations of Christ on the cross, both of which gave people the idea that the sex organs should be covered with a cloth. Like Jesus, people should conceal their genitals when they went before the Lord.[33]

Hagberg also describes customs connected to the idea that a corpse could rob a farm of its fertility. If there were concerns that this might happen, they could be allayed by placing a man's shirt in the coffin if the corpse was female or a woman's slip if the corpse was male.[34] The custom is not explained, but the idea seems to have been that the corpse's desire for the opposite sex would be satisfied by the garment and that the living would thus be spared. Many questions arise: what types of people would require this sort of measure after their death? Would it have been people known to have had an especially strong sex drive? This custom cannot be explained by Christian religious beliefs in the resurrection of the body, but instead it provides an example of the fact that Christian concepts did not totally dominate people's ideas. The few references to sexuality in the archival materials provide a hint of an imagined existence after death, in which things we normally associate with the living body continue on—including sexuality.

Awaiting Burial

While funeral preparations were being made, the body had to be kept somewhere. A barn or an outbuilding was often used for this purpose. In 1929, a woman from Södermanland related that people usually kept the corpse in a shed. The person taking care of the body strewed grain on the floor so rats would not gnaw on the body.[35] That same year, a man from the province of Närke said that in addition to a hymnal, a slice of bread was laid on the deceased's breast to discourage rats from chewing on the body.[36] Reports of how people tried to stave off attacks by rats are rare in the literature, despite the fact that the problem was probably well-known. This likely reflects the interviewers' interest in recording customs perceived to be charged with meaning rather than merely practical ones. It was also common to strew chopped spruce twigs and needles on the floor of the corpse room, which possibly had some effect against rats and bad odors.[37]

Placing a container of water in the corpse room was another way to keep the room fresh.[38] It was likely believed that the water would purify the air. The smell of corpses must have been troublesome in rooms with no means of cooling. One single respondent, a woman born in 1868, told of the use of disinfectant agents in this context:

> When someone had died, they were kept at home the entire time until the day of burial. The corpse might be at home so long that it began to smell bad before it was buried. So people put Lysol in the corpse shed and in the coffin so that it would smell better.[39]

Another way to control the smell of corpses was to dip glowing hot pieces of iron in a bucket of pine tar so the air was filled with tar-scented smoke.[40] When an old fisherman in the province of Bohuslän died in 1935, blocks of ice were placed around the bier to slow "the changing and decay of the corpse" during the warm August week between the times of death and burial.[41]

Those who had the means to do so could have the body embalmed to stop the process of decay from beginning before burial. Embalming did not become as popular in Sweden as it did in the United States, where it is the rule rather than the exception and where the custom of viewing the body continues to this day.[42] One of the Nordic Museum's informants maintained that wealthy persons were typically embalmed and described an experience with trans-Atlantic embalming: when a Swedish consul died during a visit to America, he was embalmed there and sent home in a coffin with a glass-covered hole through which the body could be seen.[43]

Funeral services most commonly took place outdoors at the cemetery, which reduced the risk of exposing participants to the smell of decaying corpses.[44] The problems of odor and rats, which seem distant today, were resolved as an increasing number of congregations built mortuaries (usually small stone houses), where corpses could be kept until burial. In hospitals, where deaths were occurring in increasing numbers, corpses were kept in refrigerated rooms or cellars. An undertaker from the town of Katrineholm reported that from about 1935 onward, it became increasingly common to transport the dead to mortuaries and by 1958 dead bodies were no longer kept at home, even in the countryside.[45] In Långåskans in the province of Härjedalen, however, no mortuary was erected until the 1950s, and until the end of that decade families still kept the corpse in a decorated room until the funeral day.[46] In the city of Borås, this custom had "almost disappeared," claimed an undertaker, who also observed: "On that count, as in so many other things, the cities are the predecessors, and the rural areas come along later."[47]

Casket Manufacturers and Undertakers

> In the old days, there were special women who tried to practice the job of undertaker and clothe the remains. As a rule, there was one in every parish.

The casket was then picked up at our shop, with their [sic] own transportation, and the remains placed in an outbuilding, wash house, wagon shed or similar building on the farm until the day of burial. About 15 years ago, all of the corpse-dressing ladies disappeared, when professional personnel from funeral homes came, saw and conquered.[48]

These are the words of funeral home director Oscar Aronsson of Falköping, giving a history of his field of work in 1958. Aronsson was born in 1900 and had worked as an undertaker in Västergötland province since 1927. His personal history is typical of the replies to the Nordic Museum's 1958 questionnaire about undertaking traditions. Most of the informants were born around 1900 (the oldest was born in 1886) and began their work during the 1920s or 1930s. Practices they described from earlier times were ones they had either experienced before they became members of the trade or had heard from an older colleague. The fact that their experiences do not extend farther back in time is not a problem; for the most part, they constituted the first generation of undertakers. Only the larger cities had funeral directors prior to 1900.[49]

Otherwise, very little information about the activities of undertakers is found in the archives of the Nordic Museum. There are many items concerning the fact that carpenters made coffins, women made funeral wreaths, and so on. In certain reports we glimpse transitional phases between a system in which all items needed for the funeral were made in the deceased's neighborhood and the dominant system of the late twentieth century, in which funeral directors managed all necessary preparations for a fee. For example, in 1945 a woman from Södermanland said that in the 1880s most coffins were built at home, but they could also be purchased with all the accessories. The grave clothes were made of purchased cloth and consisted of a definite number of parts: pillow, sheet, cover, shirt, gloves, and a cloth to cover the face.[50] The differences compared with older bridal grave clothes were considerable. A woman from Skåne gave a similar account: before ready-made grave clothes were available in stores, people bought cloth and sewed them by hand. The family did everything on its own.[51] A farmer from Halland stated that into the 1930s a carpenter would build "one or another coffin for the simpler folk," leaving it understood that everyone who had the means bought factory-made caskets.[52] A woman from Tierp in Uppland province related: "Now [by] about 1910, newer times had come, and in the town there was a funeral home which rented out their hearse. The wealthy farmers in the parish would hire this hearse for their funerals."[53]

According to another report, a carpenter would keep unassembled coffins of all sizes and qualities in stock. From the 1890s onward, grave clothes were also sold, although many chose to dress the deceased in a sheet and place a folded handkerchief over the face.

Back then, the coffin had to be ordered and made according to [the deceased's] measurements, and the deceased had to rest on a table until it was ready. Everything took time, and no one other than the members of that household or friends and neighbors had anything to do with it. It was the final service that a friend could offer, no undertakers or agents like now.[54]

Washing and dressing the dead was a task for someone special, carried out by "a couple of trusted women from the deceased's circle." This informant had taken part in this act herself and reflected:

Remarkable, when I think back in time, when I was still quite young and was asked to clothe several of the old ones from the neighborhood who had passed away. Now the undertakers and the "agent" are responsible even for this, and they arrange everything that has to do with funerals, if one wishes, and it's the most common way.[55]

As late as the 1950s, rural areas could have few or even no undertaking services. An eldery farmer from Härjedalen who worked as an undertaker for extra income reported in his questionnaire that in the 1930s, when he was also managing a general store, he had begun selling coffins, grave clothes, funeral wreaths, and bouquets. He offered no other services; the dressing of the dead was performed by the local midwife, friends of the deceased, or, later, the district's public nurse.[56]

Based on the undertakers' accounts, the history of their trade can be described as follows. When somebody died, the corpse was washed and dressed by the local person or persons usually called upon for such work. The coffin was ordered from a carpenter or built at the homestead. Later, a new form of business arose: coffin shops, selling partially or fully finished coffins that might be resold by storekeepers and carpenters. These manufacturers, dealers, and carpenters gradually began to sell more types of products and services and eventually took over tasks once reserved for family members. Often, the coffin maker would open a funeral home, and the coffin shop typically closed sometime later. Instead of being spread among many small coffin-making shops, manufacturing became concentrated in a few larger factories that delivered their goods to funeral homes nationwide. The services the funeral homes offered gradually expanded: they began to arrange for corpse transport and pallbearers, send out death announcements with invitations to the funeral and the wake, take care of refreshments for the guests, hire the priest and organist, and decorate the grave, the coffin, and the church. In addition, they assisted in clothing the deceased.

These developments proceeded quickly and took on various forms in different parts of the country. Stockholm had only three funeral parlors in the 1880s, but by the turn of the twentieth century there were more than ten. These businesses were unable to satisfy the demand for funeral services, however, and funeral arrangements were also made by church clerks and janitors, as well as by janitors at the hospitals, according to one of the city's undertakers.[57] Funeral parlors were also established in other cities and eventually in rural areas as well. According to the informants, the 1940s constituted a breakthrough period for funeral directors in Sweden. Most informants claimed that the funeral parlors have handled all arrangements connected with funerals since that decade.[58]

The Swedish Association of Funeral Directors

Swedish funeral directors organized their own association in 1922. According to the constitution written in 1932, the purpose of the association was to

> unite the undertakers (funeral homes) of Sweden, and thereby work for the improvement of their conditions and of the Swedish funeral system; to be a gathering and unifying organ for the nation's members; to be of benefit and assistance to members in the conduct of their work, through meetings and other suitable means; to encourage a sound culture of funerals and grave-care in Sweden; as well as to contribute to the strengthening of respect for the dead.[59]

How the group intended to achieve the two last goals is not evident from the constitution or from the association's other printed materials. Undoubtedly, the funeral directors wanted to be associated with "a sound culture of funerals" and "respect for the dead," but the main reason the association was established was to serve the directors' economic interests. The constitution's rhetoric is typical of the way a professional group legitimizes its field of work.

Internal conflicts were a recurrent problem for the association, as revealed in the annual reports, meeting minutes, and flyers. Replies to the questionnaires show that undertakers worried about the intense competition within the field. Some believed the association had helped to alleviate this situation, and others felt the problem remained largely unchecked.[60] An addendum to the constitution exposes the nature of the problem. A clause was added stating that the association would "by every means seek to work against bribery (gifts) and corruption within our field, and thereby seek to bring about better, more loyal working methods in the same."[61]

Funeral home director Aronsson was more explicit on this point when he wrote: "Despite keen competition [pursued by means of] bribes, which unfortunately continue, to nurses, janitors, deacons, and others, we have increased our sales each year. These conditions should be exposed, so that funeral costs may be reduced."[62] Because hospital personnel and others recommended certain firms over others, inequalities were created within the market. Perfectly legal contracts were also drawn up between particular funeral homes and the police, who used those firms when a corpse had to be taken care of in the event of an accident, suicide, or homicide.[63]

In 1932, when the association had existed for ten years, the membership was only 117, although the number of funeral homes in Sweden was estimated at around 500.[64] In that year's annual report, members were challenged to "work for increased membership." The following year the number of members had risen to 270. An Association of Funeral Product Sellers and Manufacturers (Begravningsbranschens Grossist- och Fabrikantförening) was also established, which cooperated with the funeral directors' association. Together, they sought expressly to make working conditions for non-member undertakers and manufacturers more difficult and to prevent the establishment of new funeral homes in areas where current members were already working.[65] Was this designed to keep the prices of goods and services high?[66] The association's ability to affect opportunities for a new funeral director was confirmed by an undertaker from Lidköping, who maintained that he was denied membership in the association and that the local coffin retailer worked against him. He was not granted access to materials and knowledge and thus was unable to start his own firm until he had established a cooperative relationship with a manufacturer.[67] One of the earliest members of the Swedish Association of Funeral Directors wrote that from the beginning, the association saw to it that only retailers with the right to sell to the public were allowed to become members: "The hind-ends of hospital janitors, that widespread system of weeds, were not allowed to join."[68]

A remarkable passage in the 1931 annual report can perhaps be understood in the context of the earlier discussion. Its obscure, mystifying formulations probably refer to the difficulties faced in getting people to forsake the old traditions, open their wallets, and let the undertakers do the job:

> The greatest difficulties the practitioners of this field have faced and still do face are the very limited circumstances, which are completely unaffected by all advertising or other means. This has been pointed out so many times that it should now be unnecessary to point it out yet again. It is, however, against this background that our work must be viewed.
>
> These difficulties have existed longer than the Association has existed, and this is why as soon as the Association was founded, one of its first tasks became to effect a change upon them, if possible.[69]

Ways to achieve a change in people's thinking were discussed at the association's meetings. Looking back on this situation from our time, when funeral parlors are regularly called in to make funeral arrangements, the association was obviously successful in its endeavors. Certainly, the undertakers' united effort was not the only reason funeral arrangements from the 1940s onward in Sweden were managed entirely by hired professionals. Other conceivable factors include the increased prosperity of the general populace—more people were able to pay for the services of an undertaker. Further, the fact that an increasing number of people moved around the country, often from rural areas to larger settlements, meant that the system of the exchange of goods and services between friends and neighbors diminished in importance.

There was also perhaps no reason to hold on to old customs for their own sake if family members could be spared some of the tasks that could be both physically and mentally difficult to bear and if the deceased could still be given as dignified a farewell as possible. Often, what was conceived to be dignified was also that which was modern and which could be bought for money, in contrast to the old, which involved using traditional methods of handcraft. In all events, the development and establishment of the system of funeral homes should be regarded as part of the great pattern of cultural and social change usually referred to as modernization.

One effect of the cooperation between manufacturers and funeral directors was that local differences among funerals' outward forms diminished. The products funeral parlors sold became similar throughout the entire country, as did the services they offered. Thus, local customs and traditions weakened as family members increasingly delegated the authority over death and burial to undertakers by purchasing their services. Hagberg mentions that a funeral director in 1915 corrected a family who wanted to dress a fourteen-year-old girl as a bride—it was not appropriate to do so, according to the director. Instead, she should be clothed in her confirmation dress.[70] One funeral director related that he had set families on the right track when they wanted to organize the funeral in a way that, according to him, was outmoded:

> One may at times meet with certain ideas concerning the ways in which the deceased should be cared for. In all likelihood it is usually elderly people [illegible word] not been able to "follow along with the times," who may present antiquated suggestions. Once it has been explained to them that this is not possible in modern times, they accept "the new ways."[71]

For one undertaker from Borås who reflected on funeral traditions, it was obvious that customs were in a steady state of flux. He also conveyed the sense that undertakers and funeral homes played a key role in the modernization of traditions and customs. A number of local customs survived into the 1950s, and although funeral directors had to accept them, nothing was static:

> The residents of the parish have seen this arrangement used for all of the funerals in their church, and are careful to preserve this tradition, even if many times it came about by coincidence back in the day when funerals were taken care of without the assistance of a funeral director. In the long term, the traditions surrounding funerals are the objects of a constant process of development, which

has occurred at an ever more rapid pace since even those in country areas have begun to rely upon professionals.[72]

Division of Labor

In the old Swedish peasant culture, the tasks of preparing a body prior to a funeral were usually distributed between the sexes (although there were exceptions). The women washed, clothed, and decorated the body, while the men shaved, trimmed, and carried it. In addition, the men built coffins and dug graves. This distribution basically followed the general cultural patterns involving the division of labor between the sexes.

In two paintings, Finnish artist Juho Rissanen depicted the handling of dead bodies in a rural milieu, representing the tasks as gender-specific. The paintings were created during a period in the early 1900s when Rissanen devoted himself to portrayals of everyday life and work in the impoverished milieu in which he grew up in eastern Finland.[73] In one painting (see figure 24), a powerful, serious-looking older woman is washing a male corpse that lies naked on a simple wooden plank. Next to her are a bucket of water and a piece of soap. Her grip on the stiff arm of the deceased is firm and determined as she carefully washes it with a cloth. Two women stand nearby, singing from a hymnal. The window is hung with pieces of white cloth, and in front of it on a sideboard stand several glass bottles that perhaps contain medicines (or possibly something used to prepare the body). In the center of the painting, behind the dead man, stand two men who seem to be deep in conversation. The men seem entirely outside the sphere of the women's engagement at the bier. In the other picture, fur-clad men carry a dead man on a stretcher across a snowy farmyard (see figure 26). Here the men are active while the women stand by: one cries and hugs a child; another stands watching in a doorway.[74]

Even at funeral homes, washing and dressing corpses were initially jobs for women. Some dressing-women worked for a specific funeral home, while others were employed by different firms when needed. Some informants maintained that this division of labor was eventually forsaken and that anyone at a funeral home could clothe the deceased.[75] Those who made this claim felt it was an indication of the increased level of professionalization within the funeral industry. The gender-specific division of labor within funeral homes followed several interesting patterns. Other than dressing, the tasks viewed as suitable women's jobs were general office duties and customer service in the funeral home office, while the men did the bookkeeping, drove the hearses, and served as pallbearers. Most striking is the fact that it was always the men who represented the firm outside the funeral home and were present at funerals.

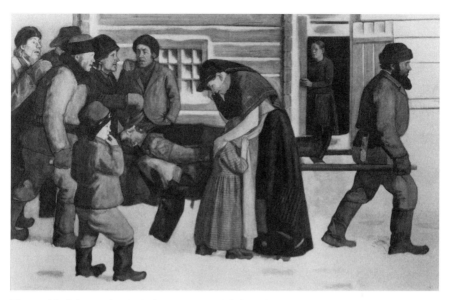

Figure 26. Watercolor by Juho Rissanen (1903) titled *A Childhood Memory*. The scene probably depicts Rissanen's father being carried home after he froze to death while ice fishing. The painting is owned by the Budapest Museum of Art. From the Photo Archives, Nationalmuseum, Stockholm.

The funeral director was usually a man.[76] The archives of the Nordic Museum, however, do reveal examples of funeral homes operated by women. Just as a carpenter might branch out into the funeral business, a seamstress or florist could increase her income by opening a funeral home. The florist would also make the flower arrangements for the funeral. One informant described two women who were seamstresses and who operated a funeral home in the town of Katrineholm. They also made artificial wreaths for use as casket decorations, sewed mourning clothes, and made mourning hats.[77]

Theologist Anna Davidsson Bremborg has studied the division of tasks between the sexes at Swedish funeral homes around the turn of the twenty-first century. She stated that the field had been dominated by men but that later, women took their place within it, and not just as office secretaries.[78] Bremborg identified two different strategies in the organization of work at funeral homes: specialization and continuity. The strategy of specialization means each employee at a funeral home takes on different tasks. In most cases, specialization is accompanied by a division of labor between the sexes. The women manage the office work and contact with the families, while the men transport and prepare the bodies and represent the firm outside the office. At funeral homes that employ the strategy of continuity, the employees divide up customers among themselves, and each carries out all the necessary tasks. Women are often shut out of this branch of work with the explanation that the job includes physically demanding tasks. Bremborg has noted that the work of collecting and transporting bodies and the tasks in the funeral ceremony spaces are perceived as manly and thus as less suitable for women.

Bremborg's study thus supports my observation that the care of the dead body was masculinized in Sweden. Around 1900, as we have seen, the jobs of washing and clothing the corpse were generally carried out by women in the home of the deceased. Clothing and placing the body in the casket then became tasks carried out by men in mortuary facilities.[79] At the same time, the history of the establishment of funeral homes can be regarded as the history of a shift in the meanings of a dead body. Whereas previously it had been important to prepare the dead body with care and make it beautiful for viewing, in recent times it seems to have become more important to haul it off and hide it in a hygienic, refrigerated storage room. Dead bodies are thus now separated from the sphere of the living in a more obvious way: through placement in a mortuary.

Customs Old and New

In her article on the washing of corpses, Ulrika Wolf-Knuts concluded that the practice served a number of purposes.[80] Through washing, impurity was removed from the body in both a symbolic and a practical/hygienic sense. The deceased was to be clean in his or her new life on the other side, both bodily and spiritually. Water, with its purifying and renewing powers, was helpful in achieving this goal. Washing also had several social aspects. It was a "labor of love," a way for survivors to show their respect for the deceased. The act also provided a form of contact between the living and the dead, as well as continuity over time. For the deceased person, washing also meant that he or she became a member of the congregation of the dead and could rest in peace. In addition, washing was a way of making certain death had occurred and that this was not a case of "premature death." Finally, washing also had aesthetic aspects: the body had to be made beautiful in preparation for the final farewell, dressed up as if for a celebration; therefore, it should be clean and handsome.[81]

This analysis can be extended to include other traditional customs and practices. If customs regarding death and burial are considered rites of passage, then washing, dressing, laying the body in the coffin, and burial all function as ways of definitely yet gradually separating the deceased from the world of the living. While all these rituals can be perceived as acts of respect (or love) for the deceased, they also have practical and social aspects. A central function of rites that are repeated again and again in the same way is to create a context, a sense of belonging and continuity in time and space. The aesthetic aspects can also be observed throughout all the rites involved in the funeral ritual as a whole, from dressing the corpse to mourning clothes and grave decorations.

The rise of undertakers and funeral parlors has been characterized as a professionalization of death.[82] The undertakers' practices are then perceived as fundamentally different from traditional customs and less imbued with meaning. Yet people's need to create meaning in death and in the dead body could not have disappeared with the advent of modernity. Would it not then be advantageous to view the work of undertakers as charged with meaning to the same degree as the older, traditional customs?

I argue that funeral practices still function as rites of passages that separate the deceased person from the world of the living and introduce him or her into that of the dead. The acts themselves have changed in form, as have the notions about them, but their overarching function is the same. The fact that washing and dressing the dead body, laying it in the coffin, transporting it, and similar functions are handled by professional service personnel does not make the ritual element disappear. For those who carry out these acts, they are part of their daily work. At the same time, for the survivors these acts are rituals that bring the deceased person's time on earth to a close.

Turning the dead over to the professional care of a funeral home is thus an *addition* to the funeral ritual rather than a *loss* of ritual. This shift can be viewed as a new type of act of love, a new way of showing respect for the dead, in which the undertaker's skills are a valued part. Even the cost of the funeral home's services can be viewed as symbolic: the deceased is worth the expense. The continuity-creating effect of funeral rites remains, but now the funeral director is the unifying leader of these rites. In an era of great social mobility, the undertaker's knowledge may also be a guarantee that everything is done the right way and that social etiquette is upheld.

The aesthetic side of death customs is, as in other ritual contexts, important and filled with meaning. Dressing and decoration are parts of the ritual acts and cannot be separated from the others. The history of the changing ways of handling the bodies of the dead is a history of changing aesthetic traditions. In Sweden, the custom of saying farewell to the deceased in the decorated corpse room or at the open coffin disappeared during the twentieth century. Yet despite the fact that funeral parlor personnel may be the only people who see the deceased, bodies are still dressed and laid in prepared caskets. The dressing of the corpse and decoration of the interior of the casket, despite their invisibility, have thus retained a ritual importance and are part of the aesthetic whole encompassing the customs of death. The flower arrangements, the design of the casket, and the decoration of the ritual room (in Sweden, most often a church, chapel, or crematorium) have, however, come to be the chief bearers of aesthetic values for participants in the funeral ritual.

The most obvious difference modern society exhibits in the handling of dead bodies and in funeral customs compared with earlier eras is one of simplification: the ritual acts have become fewer and less differentiated.[83] This simplification implies a change in people's conceptions: if the dead are no longer thought to continue living a bodily life after death, the living need not help them through acts designed to provide a good start in their new existence or to prevent them from coming back and causing damage. This simplification and the increased uniformity of both funerals and gravesites can also be viewed as part of Swedish society's aspirations toward social equality during most of the twentieth century. They are also aligned with the aesthetic and ethos of modernity, with its ideals of functionalism, minimalism, and rationalization.

In addition, the customs surrounding death have been compressed in time and space: when the deceased was washed and kept in the home; when the coffin was followed by a long procession to the cemetery, carried to the grave, and lowered into it; the family was there, close to the deceased throughout the rites. When the dead body came to be cared for by hospital employees and funeral home workers, the ritual space and ritual time were limited to the funeral itself. The dead body, previously visible at the center of these rites, was now hidden in a closed casket.

Funerals, Gender, Ethnicity, and Class

Funerals, like other customs and celebrations, were organized differently depending upon the social and cultural status of the deceased. The deceased's gender was also emphasized in several ways. For example, the ringing of church bells when somebody died indicated both gender and class status through the time of day at which the bells were rung, which of the church's bells were used, and how long they were rung.[84] The clothing and accessories that accompanied the deceased in the coffin were chosen to signal gender and age, in accordance with local customs. The ethnographic reports also indicate that experiences of death and burial were gendered. Male respondents usually described how coffins were built and carried to the cemetery, how graves were dug, and the ways church bells were rung. The women's reports contain more information about contributions to the meal at the funeral party, how the corpse was dressed, and how the room in which the corpse lay was decorated. Each sex carried out these tasks in accordance with mutual, gender-specific divisions of labor.

Class and economic resources also influenced the way the corpse looked in its coffin. Someone who was wealthy and had a strong position in society could have a more elaborate funeral than a person who was poor. In an article on working-class funerals in Gothenburg, ethnologist Birgitta Skarin Frykman has shown that it was important that the funeral was perceived as "honorable" and that it did not have the character of a pauper's funeral.[85] Social

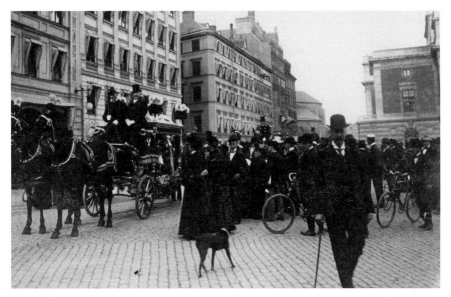

Figure 27. Funeral procession passing through the crowds in Gustaf Adolf Square, Stockholm, 1901. Stately hearses and decorations for the black horses could be rented from livery companies. Photograph by Anton Blomberg. Stockholm City Museum.

position could be shown in many ways. For example, laborers and farmers were buried during general burial hours, that is, prior to the Sunday church service. Funerals of the wealthy were held indoors in the church, while those of the less well-to-do were held in the cemetery. A bishop might conduct the funeral of high-status members of the congregation, while a local pastor led services for common folk.[86] It was at funerals of the rich that the first specialized, horse-drawn hearses were used to carry the coffin from the home to the church cemetery. In rural areas, the wealthy were the first to purchase ready-made coffins, grave clothes, and special coffin decorations.[87]

The materials on death and burial in the archives of the Nordic Museum deal almost exclusively with the customs of people who today would be referred to as ethnic Swedes. Local and regional differences are emphasized by the organization of the materials according to province and parish (rather than, for example, by the period during which they were reported or other possible methods of organization). What emerges from these materials is a "Swedish" Sweden, characterized by a rather uniform folk culture without significant class differences. The material appears in this way because those who collected it were driven by the ideas that there was an ancient "Swedish" folk culture and that it had to be documented because it risked being destroyed by the upheavals of the modern era. In this way, ethnographers participated in the construction of Swedish-ness.[88]

The Sámi of Lapland, with their particular minority culture, are represented but set apart in the archive. The material gives no systematic evidence of any other ethnic groups or systems of belief except the Protestant Christianity of the Swedish Lutheran state church. Not even the funerals of the Free Church movement are recorded.[89] This is a significant lacuna, since funerals within religious congregations other than the Swedish state church did in fact occur in Sweden (for instance, Jewish congregations have had the right to practice their own funeral rituals in designated places ever since the eighteenth century).[90]

A somewhat different picture begins to take shape when one studies the undertakers' replies to the questionnaires, however. The funeral homes did in fact arrange funerals for dead persons from other countries and of other religions. Roman Catholic as well as Jewish and Greek Orthodox funerals are mentioned in the material. Among other details, these funerals reportedly differed from Protestant services in that the coffin was open during the funeral ceremony, and the deceased lay fully clothed in the coffin under a blanket of thin fabric.[91] For one undertaker from Jönköping, a center of the evangelical revival movement, the reference to Free Church milieus was obvious. Several undertakers further mentioned that they had arranged Roma (then called Gypsy) funerals, which had their own ritual details.[92]

Patterns of class and gender also changed during the transition from traditional to modern customs. What is clear is that the numerous ways of expressing status differences in older funeral customs were replaced with greater simplicity, and funerals became more and more alike. The undertakers claim to have treated everyone the same, but those claims should be taken with skepticism; they nonetheless do point out a trend toward reducing class differences within the context of funerals. According to Oscar Aronsson of Falköping, his firm treated people of different social backgrounds the same; differences in economic status were exhibited primarily in the choice of casket. Seth Källströmer of Norsjö in the northern province of Västerbotten maintained that the poor funerals of older days were on the way out, and that there were no longer any differences in the funerals of those from different social groups and ages or between those in urban and rural areas. Edvin Walfrid Gustafsson of Katrineholm wrote in 1958:

> In death, differences of a social character no longer [exist]. Cemetery plots here are free, and all the same for everyone; grave digging, the organist, the [chapel] facility, and cremation are all free; gravestones may not be higher than 60 cm. above the ground—the same for everybody.[93]

Previously, fees had been charged for each of the services Gustafsson mentioned. The Church of Sweden also contributed to making death more egalitarian by abolishing funeral fees for members of the congregation and using the same rules for everyone (for example, holding all funeral services, not just those for members of the upper class, inside the church). It is not a historical coincidence that the concept of equality in death was supported by both funeral directors and the church because the twentieth-century Swedish Social Democratic ideal of the "People's Home" (Folkhemmet) extended into the realm of death. Nor is it surprising that the issue of class differences was of interest to the person who composed the 1958 questionnaire (Anna-Maja Nylén), while gender, class, and ethnicity were not important to ethnographers of the early 1900s.

The new simplicity in funerals was, however (at least during the first half of the twentieth century), an indicator of division between the social classes. It was primarily the upper classes who chose simplicity, as church historian Hilding Pleijel has shown in his book *Jordfästning i stillhet: Från samhällsstraff till privatceremoni*. A revealing summary of this development was given by a funeral home director from Värnamo:

> What has changed the most in the last 35 years is that you can no longer judge the social standing or wealth of the deceased based on his final earthly journey. The funerals for people from the public old-age homes are as a rule just as dignified and expensive as a bank director's. The latter's funeral is often simpler than that of the former.[94]

The leveling of differences evidenced in the questionnaire material seems not to have taken place until well into the twentieth century, however. In the 1930s, it was still a point of honor for laborers and rural people to prepare the deceased for burial themselves, according to an undertaker from the town of Alvesta. People of "somewhat better standing," on the other hand, did not want to be bothered with such tasks.[95]

The reports described in this chapter point in the same direction as many others: the first people to use the services of funeral homes were city-dwelling members of the upper classes, but during the first half of the twentieth century the new patterns spread to groups throughout the country. An entirely new way of preparing the dead body for the grave was established by the 1940s: preparations were handled by a corps of male professionals rather than by women close to the deceased, who followed tradition-determined customs. Handling the dead body had become more a matter of hygiene, budget concerns, and reverence than of close bodily contact and magic. The modern rites of passage surrounding death and burial more strongly emphasized separation, drawing strict boundaries between living and dead bodies.

When corpses were still laid out for viewing before the funeral, they were often photographed, either on the death bed or in the casket. This practice had begun with the introduction of photography in the 1840s. The death portrait is a centuries-old genre that was renewed with the use of modern technology. Chapter 5 examines this photographic practice.

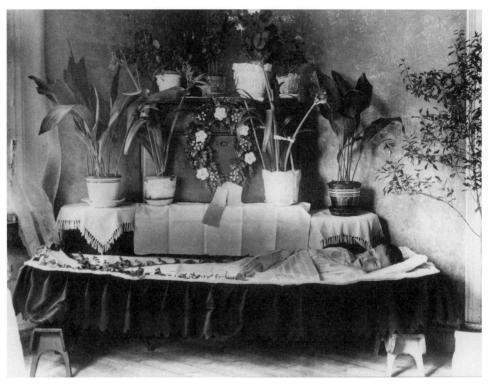

Figure 28. A boy of sixteen laid out in an open casket on the island of Orust, 1901 (photographer unknown). Photographic Collection, Nordic Museum, Stockholm.

Chapter Five

Picturing the Dead

In a photograph from 1901, a dead boy lies in a coffin (see figure 28). The boy's head rests on a pillow and is turned toward the photographer so the facial features can be clearly seen. His shirt is pleated, and so is the sheet with which he is covered. His right hand rests on top of the sheet in a somewhat awkward position, and inside the coffin various types of leaves are arranged like a garland. The coffin stands upon two stools and has been decorated with dark fabric folded around its edges. Behind it, potted plants are arranged on small tables covered with pressed linens. There is also a dresser with an artificial-looking wreath of flowers decorated with ribbons. The plants are placed symmetrically, with the wreath as the centerpiece. Everything is carefully arranged in the corner of a simple-looking room with a plain wooden floor. Part of a door frame is visible to the right, as is a large tree-like plant. To the left is a white lace curtain by a window from which daylight softly falls.

The photograph was taken in the village of Fiskebäckskil in the province of Bohuslän, and the boy, whose name was Anders, was sixteen years old when he died. The photographer is unknown, but very few people in the country owned cameras at that time, so the photographer was likely a local professional.[1]

Quite a few pictures of this type have been preserved from the years around the turn of the twentieth century. They were taken in rural as well as urban milieus, and the scenes they depict range from the deathbeds of royalty and celebrities to the simple funerals of the poor. Many, like the picture of Anders, show a dead person in a coffin surrounded by decorations, while others focus more on the funeral guests and decorations than on the deceased. There are also pictures of closed coffins, funeral processions, funeral services in churches or in cemeteries, the lowering of coffins into graves, and similar motifs. People wanted to commemorate death, much as we keep pictures of weddings and other celebrations and events today.

These pictures seem foreign to a present-day viewer, which make them interesting research objects. To make sense of this photographic genre and its rise and fall, I will discuss it within the context of photographic history. I have studied Swedish photographs in the image archives of the Nordic Museum and of the Stockholm City Museum and selected items according to a few rather loose criteria, mainly that at least one of these details about each photo can be identified: the name of the photographer, the name of the deceased, a geographic area, or a specific year. I have also tried to represent different types of photographs, using commonly occurring types rather than particularly imaginative or artistic photos.[2] The focus of my analysis is on the visual representation of the dead and the cultural history of this photographic practice in relation to the modernization of Sweden.

A Re-Formed Genre of Portraiture

The custom of photographing deceased persons is as old as photography itself. In the mid-1800s, the novel photographic technology was employed to renew an old visual genre: the death portrait. Photographers adopted existing traditions of portraiture and adapted them to the new medium. At the same time, they made portraits available to people who had never had the means to have a portrait made.[3] Since at least the sixteenth century, kings and other prominent people had been portrayed in death.[4]

The first member of the Swedish royal family to be photographed after death was King Oskar I, who died in 1859. The widowed Queen Josefina gave copies of the photo to her children and their spouses as a memento of the day of the king's death. At least two of her children hung the photograph of their dead father in their bedrooms. In the picture, the king, with his hair neatly combed, lies in a bed supported by thick pillows, with his hands on top of the covers. Despite the modern technology used to produce the picture, the photographer drew upon the long-established tradition of painted or drawn deathbed portraits of deceased rulers. When Oskar I was photographed on his deathbed, a new tradition was introduced into the royal house. Photography became the royal family's favorite form of death portraiture.[5]

In the succeeding decades, this practice spread to middle-class circles. Thanks to increasingly inexpensive methods of photography, many soon had the opportunity to memorialize their loved ones in this way. Even in isolated rural areas, it became possible to create portraits the dead when photographers took up business in small towns and made house calls. Photographs of the poor often show the deceased lying in their coffins. By contrast, wealthy or royal persons were shown either lying in a bed (i.e., on their deathbed) or lying in state, after the body had been dressed and put on display in a decorated room (see figure 29).

In Sweden, little has been written about this genre of photography. Photographs of the deceased are sometimes used as illustrations in ethnographic texts about customs and traditions surrounding death and burial, as in Louise Hagberg's *När döden gästar*. In these contexts, the genre is not discussed; rather, the pictures are used as visual evidence of particular customs, such as the how the deceased were clothed or how corpse rooms were decorated.[6]

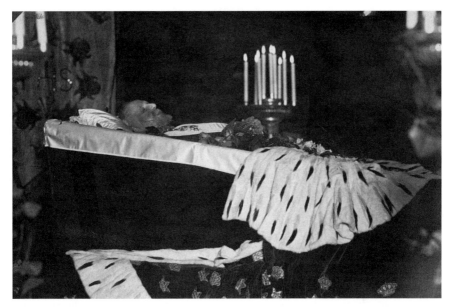

Figure 29. The body of King Oscar II lying in state, wearing formal dress and with an ermine mantle draped over the casket. Photograph by Oscar Ellqvist, 1907. Stockholm City Museum.

Photographic images of the dead are also found in photo-historic works as examples of a particular photographer's work or of the milieus or photographic genres of days gone by, but the genre itself is not discussed. The pictures occur more as a type of exotic artefact from the dawn of photography or as illustrations of outmoded customs.[7]

On the international scene, a small number of books and articles have been published on the subject, beginning in the mid-1980s. This type of photograph seems to have gone unnoticed until recent years. The scholars working in this field come from Denmark, Iceland, the Netherlands, and United States, which indicates that the genre was widespread in Western culture.[8] The most comprehensive study is by American anthropologist Jay Ruby, who in *Secure the Shadow: Death and Photography in America* analyzes a vast number of images, in combination with written sources, and interviews photographers and private users.

Funeral Reporting

Reports from funerals were much more common in Swedish illustrated weeklies around the turn of the twentieth century than they are in the media today. Sweden's daily newspapers also published reports from the funerals of nationally known individuals. Images of funeral processions, memorial stones, and decorated coffins often illustrated notices or articles about notable persons who had passed away. For the 1901 funeral of Artur Hazelius, founder of the Skansen open-air museum in Stockholm, the magazine *Hvar 8 Dag* ran a three-page report with eight pictures.[9] That same year magazines also gave extensive coverage to the funerals of Arctic explorer and geographer A. E. Nordenskiöld and the German Empress Victoria, widow of Kaiser Friedrich III. Less well-known persons were also featured, such as Swedish society matron Lilly Bäckström and a General Bergman. In the case of Bergman, photos showed the military honors that were held as he lay in state, and in Bäckström's case they showed the decorations around her grave site, "the beautiful place where the beloved lady now rests in final peace."[10] In general, fewer women's funerals were reported, and the language in the reports is clearly characterized by gendered conventions. Gender differences are less obvious in the images: the German empress's catafalque was flanked by members of the military, and Nordenskiöld's was surrounded by flowers.[11] However, none of these pictures shows the deceased person: the coffins are closed, and it is the social events occurring around them or the decorative flourishes that are represented.

When an especially prominent person died, the reports of his or her death and funeral could continue for several weeks. Following the death of King Oscar II in December 1907, *Hvar 8 Dag* ran one edition almost entirely devoted to the king's memory, and the three successive editions contained pictures of him lying in state, his funeral procession, committal service, and interment.[12] In the December 15 edition, the magazine ran two pictures under the heading "The Nation in Grief and Sorrow." The lower one is a photograph of "The Crowd Outside the Castle a Few Hours after the King's Death." The upper picture, which has a thin, black frame, is a photograph that, according to the caption, shows "the King upon His Deathbed." (see figure 30). It is not a photo of the final moments of Oscar II's life but rather one of his dead body, arranged for the photo. The king lies in a luxuriously made bed, dressed in his nightshirt, with his hands clasped over his breast. There is no doubt that he is dead—there are roses in the bed, and chrysanthemums are effectively arranged against the black background.

This photo adheres to the conventions of the genre. The style is serene, since the subject of the picture is a member of the royal family. Figure 31 is completely different. This photo was presumably shot at the same time but from a different angle, creating a scene that differs markedly from the ceremoniousness of the first picture. The king looks somewhat ruffled and unkempt, and his entire body is covered with a confusion of flowers. The flowers in and around the bed look somewhat wilted. This photograph, extraordinarily, documents the overall arrangement or production of the

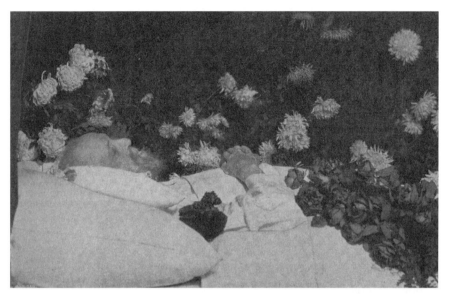

Figure 30. The official photograph of the dead King Oscar II on his deathbed. Photograph by [Ernest] Florman, *Hvar 8:e Dag* (December 12, 1907): 123. Duplication: Kungl. biblioteket - National Library of Sweden.

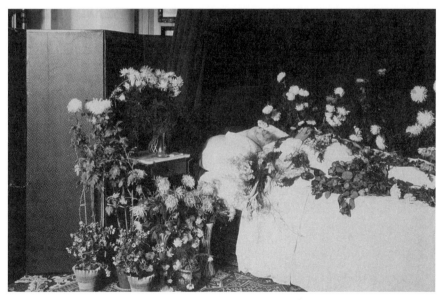

Figue 31. Oscar II on his deathbed, photographed from a different angle, showing more of the arrangement of the room (1907, photographer unknown). Stockholm City Museum.

entire scene rather than focusing on the king's person. The upper left corner of the photo provides a glimpse of a corner of the room: a tiled stove and a few framed pictures on the wall are visible. Otherwise, the room has been prepared for the photography session with a folding screen and a thick, black, ribbon-hemmed drapery behind and around the king's resting place. This photograph was never published, and why it was preserved is a mystery.

These two photographs differ markedly. The first is carefully staged, displaying a high degree of conscious, ritualized construction. Because of its less strict composition, the second one is more usable as a source about the custom of photographing the dead and how such photo shots were arranged. Neither picture reveals what the room looked like when it was arranged for people to say farewell to the king. This should be kept in mind when viewing the pictures from rural areas later in this chapter.

The funeral of Swedish poet Gustaf Fröding was also covered extensively in *Hvar 8 Dag*. On February 19, 1911, two pages were devoted to "The Final Journey of the People's Poet."[13] The first of these two pages has a montage of two photographs framed by a drawing of drapery and a lyre, the symbol of poetry (see figure 32). The larger of the photographs is a portrait taken during Fröding's illness, depicted in the form of a medallion. Below it is a photo from the poet's "death room," with Fröding in a coffin, dressed in a simple shirt, with his head on a pile of pillows and his hands on the covers. There are palms at his head, flowers are arranged in and around the coffin, and a fanciful candelabrum is fairly close to the coffin. The photo does not depart from the conventions of the genre in any way, not in the arrangement of the room, the arrangement of the corpse, or the composition of the picture itself. It is as conventional an image as one could expect from a weekly magazine of that era.

The photo was likely taken by Axel Malmström, well-known for his depictions of Stockholm, who often worked for *Hvar 8 Dag*. Some of Malmström's pictures from the same occasion are entirely different. The composition of one of them is typical for this genre, but Malmström has moved closer to the coffin and recorded the scene in a different way (see figure 33). In this photo, other forces than the conventions of the press seem to have been at work. The photographer seems more interested in portraying the human being lying there and in capturing the interplay of light in the room. The sharp winter sunlight comes in through windows outside the picture and shines on the top of the dead man's head and hands. Even the palm leaves are vivified by the light, and a blooming lilac bush is luminous. For the next picture, the photographer moved in even closer for a shot of Fröding's profile. It is a distinct and piercing portrait, at once a loving and frank picture of the dead man (see figure 34). The slanting light brings out the structure of the skin, which is dark and sunken under the eyes. The hair and beard reveal the strokes of a comb. At the same time, the interplay of light and shade

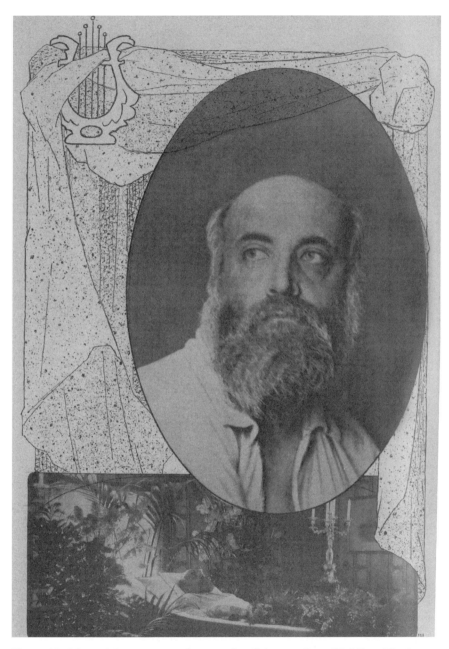

Figure 32. Memorial montage to the great Swedish poet Gustaf Fröding. The lower of the two photographs, showing the death room, was probably taken by Axel Malmström. Photographer of the first photo unknown. *Hvar 8:e Dag* (February 19, 1911): 328. Duplication: Kungl. biblioteket - National Library of Sweden.

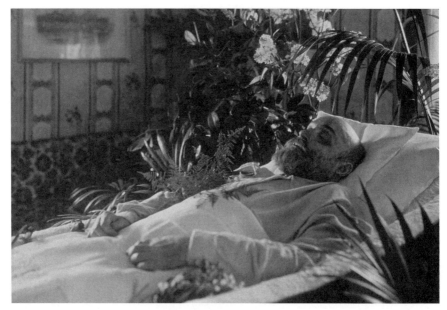

Figure 33. Death portrait of Gustaf Fröding, showing his torso and face. Photograph by Axel Malmström, 1911. Stockholm City Museum.

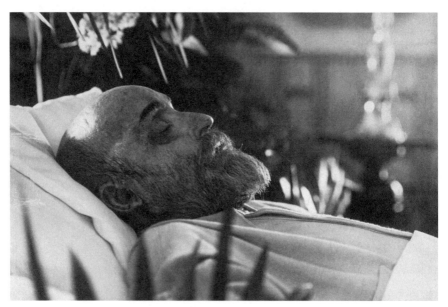

Figure 34. Close-up of Gustaf Fröding. Photograph by Axel Malmström, 1911. Stockholm City Museum.

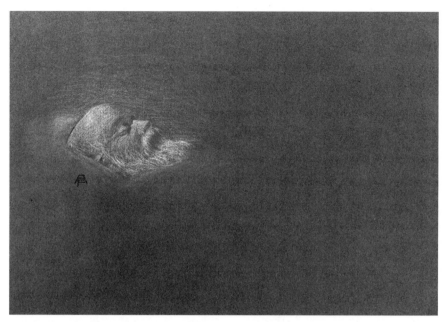

Figure 35. Chalk drawing of Gustaf Fröding, by Anders Forsberg, 1911. National Museum of Fine Arts, Stockholm, Collection of Drawings, 1956.

makes the profile glow enigmatically. The photographer thus exceeded the expectations of the genre and created a representation of death as a state of transcendence.

Yet another picture of the dead Fröding is a white chalk drawing on gray paper by artist Anders Forsberg (see figure 35). According to a slightly sarcastic note by the artist on the back of the paper, the portrait depicts "Gustaf Fröding a few hours after death on February 8, 1911. This drawing was made just before his autopsy, and the doctor was kind enough to wait fifteen minutes until it was finished."[14] Although Forsberg's drawing was made before the autopsy, the photographs were probably taken afterward, since the corpse had been put in order and the room was decorated with flowers. The photographs of Fröding thus show a dead national poet without a brain—giving these pictures another dimension.

The level of interest focused on the deceased Fröding would not have been devoted to just anyone. Fröding was a national poet who had lived a stormy life, and there was a strong desire to preserve the image of his face—so peaceful in death—in as many different media as possible: in photographs, newspaper articles, and a chalk drawing. In addition, his brain was preserved and added to the anatomical collection of the Karolinska Institute.[15]

Private Photographs of the Dead

Among the photographs of dead persons found in the photo archives of the Nordic Museum and the Stockholm City Museum, a number of types can be discerned. These pictures were composed according to certain recurring patterns, which indicates that the genre became established fairly quickly and its conventions soon became standard. The photographs fall into one of four standard types: *close-ups,* showing primarily the face of the deceased; *head-and-shoulders shots,* in which the upper body of the deceased and a little of the surroundings can be seen; *full-length shots,* showing the entire casket and its decorations and sometimes people standing next to it; and finally, *scene shots,* often taken outdoors, with the casket in the center. The scene shots often have the character of group photos, showing a large number of funeral guests. The full-length and head-and-shoulders shots outnumber the other types. The photographs are sometimes shot from above and beside the casket, but more often they are taken at a right angle to the coffin, showing the face of the deceased in profile or turned toward the photographer.

There are both indoor and outdoor photos. Those shot outside are usually from rural locations, while the environments shown in the indoor photographs vary. They span all social classes, from royal bedchambers and the parlors of nobility to simple rooms with rough plank walls. Some of the rural milieus depicted seem impoverished, although if a family chose to spend money on a photograph, they may not have been as poor as they seem. On the other hand, a photograph of this type might have been considered so significant that it was worth going without something else in order to have it. Such a picture was often the first and only photograph of a family member, especially in the case of young children.[16] Death portraits of children, youths, and older persons are more common than pictures of adults who died in middle age.

The visible parts of the dead bodies in these photographs are the face and often one or both of the hands. The rest of the body is usually covered by white clothing and a white shroud. A few atypical photos show a corpse dressed in finery. Deceased women are sometimes dressed as brides, with crowns of myrtle and veils (see figure 25). The caskets are almost always decorated with lace, ribbons, and frills. There are often flowers and leaves in the casket: myrtle, ferns, buttercups, and roses are common. Sometimes a bouquet of flowers is placed in the hands of the deceased. The room in which the casket stands is often also decorated: simply (as in figure 28) or elaborately, according to the household's social and financial situation.

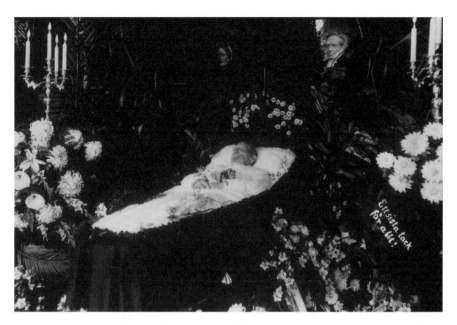

Figure 36. The ancestors of this deceased building entrepreneur watch over him from the walls, and the survivors honor him with flowers and a ribbon bearing the traditional funeral text "A final thank you for everything." Photograph by Frans Gustaf Klemming, Stockholm (undated). Stockholm City Museum.

Bourgeois Milieus

The photographs from wealthier milieus are crowded with palms, flower arrangements, wreaths with ribbons, and candelabras with live candles. The casket and its contents sometimes seem almost overlooked, as though interest in the decorations had taken precedence over them.

The decorations were especially important in bourgeois milieus. In figure 36, even the ancestors of the deceased construction company owner are included, staring down from portraits on the walls. A satin ribbon bearing the customary Swedish funeral text *Ett sista tack för allt* ("A final thank you") is arranged prominently in the foreground. This was a display of funerary honor on par with the social standing the deceased enjoyed in life. The photograph itself could also serve as a symbol of social status. Into at least the early twentieth century, the wealthier a family was, the more luxurious the funeral and the more elaborate the decorations in the death room.[17]

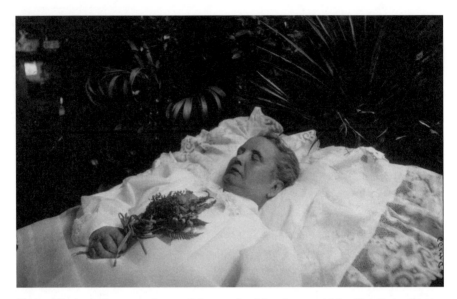

Figure 37. An intimate and peaceful portrait of the deceased Mrs. Nordkvist. Photograph by Frans Gustaf Klemming, Stockholm (undated). Stockholm City Museum.

There is also a noticeable tendency to compose the photographs according to the gender of the deceased. For a man, the photograph is more often a full-length shot, and a number of impressive wreaths bearing sentiments of praise are clearly displayed. In contrast, close-ups and head-and-shoulders shots are more common for deceased women—the person is the centerpiece, and the photograph is more of a portrait. This tendency is hardly surprising, since it follows the stereotypical conceptions of the time of men as active, extroverted, and defined by their social roles and of women as caretakers of family, home, and emotional life.

For example, compare figure 36 with the photo of the deceased Mrs. Nordkvist in figure 37. In the former, the living thank the man for contributions he made during his life, and through the portraits on the wall he is connected with history. The decorations are a display of homage to an important person. In the photograph of the woman, by contrast, her face is the most important element. Her graying hair shows that she is elderly, but her face is smooth and harmonious—and undoubtedly retouched. Bedded down in white lace, she seems to sleep in final peace. The bouquet she holds in her hand and the palms in the background indicate that this is the sleep of death. Rather than making the room more impressive, as in the photograph of the construction company owner, the palm branches frame the picture and strengthen its sense of calm.

Rural Milieus

In rural, outdoor photographs, the casket and its decorations are central—the lid, with its wreaths and ribbons, often lies beside the casket, clearly visible in the picture. However, if the family hoped to impress people with any detail, it was by the number of funeral guests. These photos were typically taken in connection with the traditional *utsjungning* (roughly translated, "the final hymn"): the funeral guests gathered at the home of the deceased to pay their final respects and sing funeral hymns before the lid of the casket was nailed in place and the procession left for the church. The pictures of this type are usually fairly similar. Here I will compare two photographs from the province of Dalarna.

The first was photographed in the village of Djura in the 1890s (see figure 38). A group of nearly thirty people is gathered in front of a farm building. The casket lid and the casket holding the deceased are in front of the group. Everyone's eyes are fixed on the deceased. Most of the women, dressed in traditional costume, are gathered to the right, and a number of them have folded hands as if in prayer. While some of the men are wearing sheepskin coats, most are dressed in dark clothing. All are wearing some sort of headgear, and they appear very serious. There is a boy among the women, the only child in the picture. The photograph is carefully arranged by the photographer.

It is understandable that photographs such as this were of interest to Swedish folklore researchers in their study of local customs and traditions. Louise Hagberg used this picture as an illustration in her chapter "When the Deceased Is Carried Out," under the heading "The Final Hymn and Farewell."[18] Hagberg does not comment on this photograph; she uses it as a silent accompaniment to the text, relying on it to speak for itself, to give visual form to the customs covered in the text—that is, gathering around the casket of the deceased to say farewell, singing a hymn, and holding a homily. The cardboard on which the photograph was mounted bears the note "*sjunga eller läsa ut*" ("singing a final hymn or reading a final prayer").

Many of the photographs of this type in the archives of the Nordic Museum also bear the note "Donated by L. Hagberg, 1913." One of the reasons these photographs exist today is because of the type of folklore research Hagberg pursued, not because this type of photograph was deemed to be of interest in and of itself. Today, it is impossible to approach these photographs in the naive way Hagberg did, taking them as true reflections of the realities of Swedish folk life. Figure 38 is a group portrait, or a staged depiction of a farewell gathering, rather than an "authentic" documentation of one. But perhaps the manufactured nature of these photographs did not matter for Hagberg and her colleagues. Is it possible that we have only recently come to regard values such as "authentic," unstaged," and "natural" as necessary prerequisites for a documentary

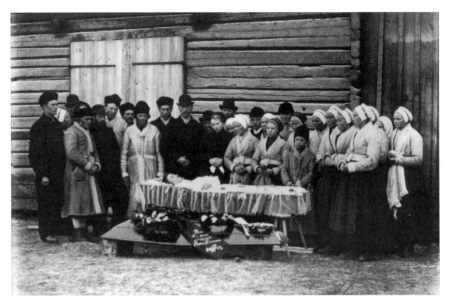

Figure 38. A carefully staged representation of a farewell gathering in the village of Djura, Dalecarlia, ca. 1900. Photograph by Hans Per Persson. Photographic Collection, Nordic Museum.

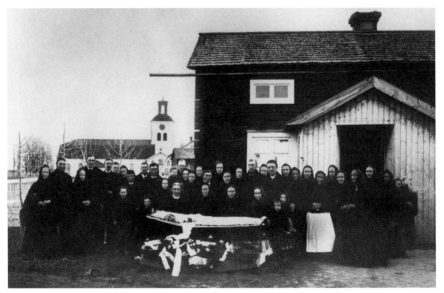

Figure 39. Group portrait of funeral guests and the deceased in front of his house, with the village church in the background, 1895. Photograph by Jonas E. Ericsson, Järna, Dalecarlia. Photographic Collection, Nordic Museum.

photograph? Could photographs that were staged "*as if*" the events were actually taking place have a completely acceptable approximate value?[19]

The second photograph was taken in the village of Järna in 1895. About forty darkly clothed persons of various ages are gathered behind an open casket in a farmyard (see figure 39). None of the men is wearing a hat, while the women and girls all wear dark kerchiefs. Most of those pictured look directly into the camera, some with a suspicious and concerned gaze, others more open and curious. The background shows a farmhouse on the right, and to the left a church can be seen a small distance away. A row of people is seated immediately behind the casket—presumably the closest family members. This photograph is also carefully composed, but it differs from the symmetrical and highly concentrated composition of figure 38. The photograph in figure 39 tells more of a story: the individual faces of the funeral guests are clearly visible; the home of the deceased is large and impressive and has a prominent place in the picture, as does the church, to which the procession will soon make its way.

Photographers in the late 1800s and early 1900s often supplemented their studio portrait work with another activity, such as photographing landscapes, rural scenes, and cityscapes. From the perspective of cultural history, some of the disappearing milieus they photographed are of even greater interest today.[20] But most of the photographs of deceased persons preserved in archives were likely commissioned by the families of the deceased, and a photographer would only occasionally have produced such photographs for other reasons.

Figure 40 might be one of these exceptions. It could also be a remarkable shot from a series. Whatever the case, it is markedly different from all other casket photos I have come across. The people photographed are not arranged in a conventional way. The deceased woman lies in her casket, bedded down in white cloth with a white kerchief on her head. The scene is austere; no flowers or other decorations beautify it or indicate the gender of the deceased. Further, her face does not reveal her gender. It is only thanks to the archival catalog that I know this is a woman, a female freeholder from the community of Utanmyra in the province of Dalecarlia. The photographer, Johan Öhman, has captured a remarkable scene with a touching mood, showing intricate relationships and complicated gazes. The man in front of the casket is looking at the deceased, with his profile to the camera. In one hand, he holds his hat, and with the other he grasps the deceased's hand. As he stands there in his ill-fitting suit, he looks simultaneously overcome with emotion and awkward. The man's exterior—with his pale forehead and sunburned face, his large, callused hands, and the crow's feet around his eyes—reveals a life of physical labor. The face of the deceased is turned toward the photographer. Directly behind the deceased's head sits an old woman in traditional costume. Her gaze is fixed on the photographer with narrowed eyes. Looking out of the window to the right, another pair of eyes meets those of the viewer. It is a small boy wearing a cap, watching the photographer at

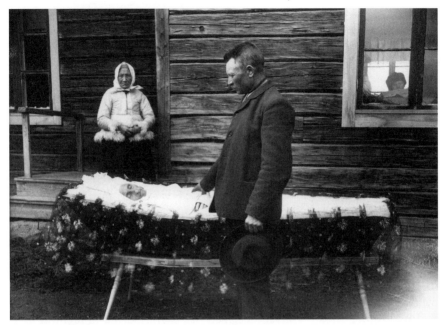

Figure 40. Open casket farewell scene from the village of Utanmyra, Dalecarlia, 1908. Photograph by John Öhman. Photographic Collection, Nordic Museum.

work. The man's relationship to the deceased is clearly the central story the photographer sought to convey. But as a viewer, I am struck by the other relationships revealed here—those among the woman, the boy, and the photographer and between the photographer and the deceased.

Images of Deceased Children

Many of the photographs found in the archives are of dead children. However, photographs of the dead bodies of children are far from dominant, contrary to what one is led to believe in an article on photographic history by Danish photo-historian Bjarne Kildegaard.[21] Circumstances may have been different in Denmark. The differences between Swedish and Danish photo collections may also have resulted from the nature of the collections themselves or from the interests or attentions of individual researchers.

While the photographs of deceased children are in many ways similar to those of adults, several characteristics differentiate them. First, there are fewer room decorations and flower arrangements in pictures of children, in both rural and bourgeois settings. The caskets, however, are sometimes very elaborate and well decorated.[22] Second, deceased children are never surrounded by large groups of people. When living people are shown in these photographs, it is always a small group consisting of the closest family members (see figures 41 and 42). I have observed no gender-based differences in the composition of these photos. A further difference is that children are often shown with open eyes and mouth. Overall, photographs of deceased children are more intimate, simpler, and focused more on the child than on the surroundings compared with photographs of dead adults. For many families, a photograph of this type would have been the first and only photograph of the child, making it especially important to display the facial features.

One unusual photograph shows a deceased young boy with a sailboat (see figure 43). The photograph is artfully arranged, and the photographer, Frans Gustaf Klemming—who was related to the boy—took several variations of this shot, both with and without the sailboat. Without the boat, this picture is just like many other photos of the same type. The inclusion of the boat introduces a symbolic dimension, however, turning the photograph into something else. The beautiful wooden model boat may have been the boy's most beloved toy. In this extremely light photograph, the placement of the boat above the boy's head gives rise to further associations. It brings thoughts of life after death and of the various mythical boats that in the afterlife carry the souls of the dead to their destination: over the River Styx, to the Island of the Dead, or across the seas of ancient Norse myths. The presence of the white sailboat's graceful hull also makes the shape of the casket seem rather boat-like: one can imagine it floating away with the boy, with the pale window curtain as a sail.

The Production and Use of Death Portraits

This section explores how photographs of dead persons were used and produced, to understand their place in the visual culture at the turn of the twentieth century.

Photographers and Death

In an article in the *Philadelphia Photographer* in 1877, photographer Charlie E. Orr provided instructions to his colleagues on how to prepare portrait photos of deceased persons. First, the body should be placed on a sofa or chaise lounge and arranged in a sitting pose, with the head and shoulders positioned to make the person look as alive as possible. Then, after lighting and camera adjustments were made, came the most important step—opening the eyes of the deceased: "this you can effect handily by using the handle of a teaspoon; put the upper lids down, they will stay; turn the eyeball around to its proper place, and you will have the face nearly as natural as

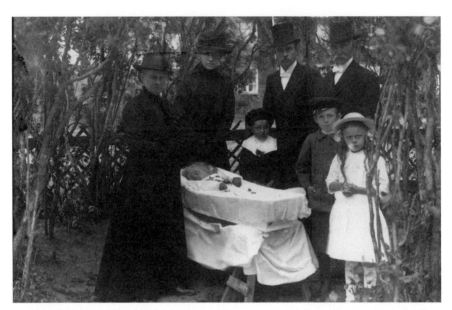

Figure 41. A little girl's casket on two sawhorses in a garden, with dressed-up family members. Photograph by Carl Ohlin, province of Värmland (undated). Photographic Collection, Nordic Museum.

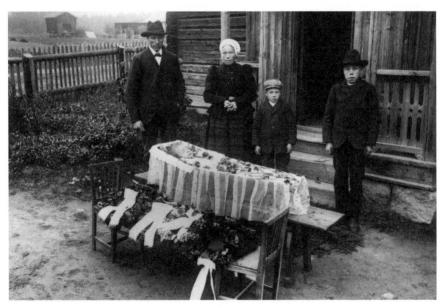

Figure 42. Even poorer families spent good money on commemorative photographs of dead children. Photograph by A. Ericsson, Dalecarlia, 1912. Photographic Collection, Nordic Museum.

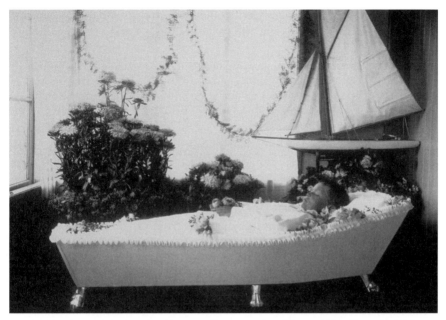

Figure 43. Evocative picture of a young boy and his sailboat, 1905. Photograph by Frans Gustaf Klemming, Stockholm. Stockholm City Museum.

life. Proper retouching will remove the blank expression and the stare of the eyes." Even though Orr seems very practical and unsentimental in his description of such work-related encounters with death, he nonetheless called photographing corpses an "unpleasant duty."[23]

I have been unable to find any similar instructions in Swedish photographic journals and handbooks from the era around the turn of the twentieth century. Perhaps experiences and advice were more often conveyed orally from one photographer to the next rather than by the written word. Or perhaps Orr's advice was not relevant to the Swedish context: photographs that presented the dead as if they were alive were common in the United States but not in Sweden. When a deceased person was to be photographed in the casket, the body had already been arranged by the funeral parlor or the family, and the photographer only needed to see to it that the face was clearly visible in the picture. Usually, the head of the deceased lay high in the casket, supported by an extra pillow, and it was often turned to the side so it could be seen better.

Undoubtedly, as the photographs prove, Swedish photographers were often hired to take portraits of the deceased, but I have only found a small number of historical narratives of such experiences. For his book on women photographers in Sweden, *Ljusets hemligheter: Kvinnligt fotografi 1861–1986*, Clas Thor interviewed ninety-five-year-old Ellen Wahlström. The stories Wahlström told about her career as a photographer in the small town of Grythyttan indicate that photographing dead people was part of everyday work:

> In our work, we followed people from the cradle to the grave. I always remember the jobs related to all the deaths as especially troublesome. During the First World War, when the influenza epidemic swept through the area, the bodies were laid out row upon row.[24]

Exactly what was troublesome about photographing the deceased was not articulated. Perhaps it was emotionally difficult, or perhaps having to meet with mourning family members was draining.

While photographs of the deceased were common, they could still be controversial. In her book *Självskrivna liv: Studier i äldre folkliga levnadsminnen*, ethnographer Britt Liljewall recounts an episode from the province of Jämtland that is of interest in this context. When his two-year-old daughter died, farmer Olof Pålsson wanted to have her photographed, but the wife of "Photographer Eriksson" said no. Liljewall's interpretation of this opposition of wills was that the photographer's wife articulated a more modern attitude toward death. Her opposition may also have stemmed from the folk belief that the making of portraits was close to idolatry.[25] In this particular case, it is impossible to determine the exact basis for the controversy. It is, however, interesting that some people found photographs of the deceased inappropriate.

Jay Ruby maintains that photographs of this type were uncontroversial in the United States during the nineteenth century. Photographing the deceased was a frequent and open cultural practice. Some years into the 1900s, the composition of the photographs changed so that the funeral or the calling hours became more important than the corpse itself. Photographs of the deceased became increasingly private in nature and were shown only in extremely limited social circles, a change he ties to the rise of amateur photography. According to Ruby, the custom of photographing the deceased survived, but it was concealed. The demand for these pictures remained but was no longer officially supported.[26]

Most of the photographs I have found in Swedish archives were taken in the decades just before and after 1900. Does this mean the genre fell out of fashion after that? It is possible that it survived longer even in Sweden but that it became invisible and private, as in the United States. Most of those who replied to the Nordic Museum's 1954 questionnaire on portrait photography did not mention photographs related to funerals, although it was a question on the list. Some answered that such photographs were never or very seldom taken.[27] These claims could mean that the custom was never especially prevalent in Sweden. Another interpretation might be that the custom had fallen into disrepute and that the informants did not want to admit they knew of it.

When interviewed in 1993, photographer Sten Didrik Bellander provided clear evidence that photographs of deceased persons continued to be taken in Sweden until the mid-twentieth century.[28] When Bellander assumed ownership of the Savoy photo studio in Stockholm in 1948, photographing the deceased was one of the firm's established specialties. According to Bellander, the previous owner had a standing relationship with a church administrative office, which would let the Savoy studio know when someone died. The photographers would telephone the survivors and offer their services. The portraits cost fifteen Swedish crowns and were often shot in a church, where the lid of the casket was removed expressly for the photographer. Bellander, a native of Stockholm, was surprised that photographs of the deceased were still made in Stockholm and that the practice was so common: "you never heard about it, but it was done." When he took over the Savoy studio, he had heard that this type of photograph was ordered only in rural areas. He does not seem to have enjoyed photographing dead persons, for as soon as his new business achieved financial stability, he stopped taking such jobs. This report shows that the practice was hidden and was dying out.

Although present-day professional photographers in Sweden may occasionally be assigned to take pictures at the funeral of a celebrity, they are almost never hired by private individuals to photograph dead family members, according to a series of telephone interviews I conducted with professional photographers in the Stockholm region in May 2000. Of those I questioned, several photographers who had long been active in the field had taken such photographs, but at the time of the interviews they had not done so for at least ten to fifteen years. The deceased individuals photographed had mostly been elderly immigrants, and the photographs were taken in a church, a chapel, or a side room at one of the same. None of the photographers interviewed had ever taken photographs of a deceased person at his or her home, and they had never photographed the body of a young person.[29]

Uses of Death Portraits

It is difficult to determine how photographs of the deceased were used by those who commissioned them. An exploration of this question would require a more thorough examination utilizing interviews, studies of letters and diaries, and searches through old photo albums and photographers' preserved collections and business ledgers. Nonetheless, there are a few indications of how these photographs were used.

First, conclusions can be drawn from the format of the photographs. When they first became widespread in Sweden in the 1860s, the most common photographic format was the calling card (*visitkort,* from the French *cartes-de-visite*). The actual image was circa 3½ × 2 inches (9 × 6 cm) and

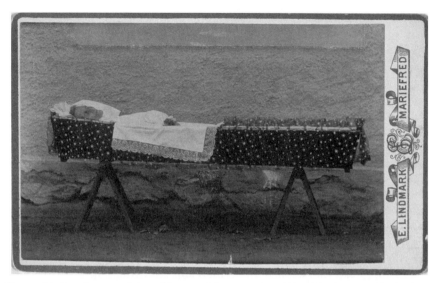

Figure 44. Death portrait in calling card format, circa 3½ × 2 inches, ca. 1896. Photograph by E. Lindmark, Mariefred, province of Södermanland. Photographic Collection, Nordic Museum.

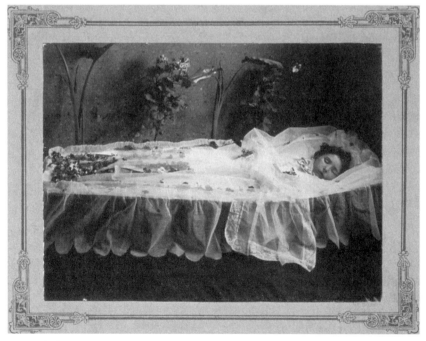

Figure 45. Small photograph mounted on a large cardboard mat. Photograph by A. Lagergren, Visby (undated, before 1905). Photographic Collection, Nordic Museum.

was mounted on cardboard, often imprinted with the photographer's name. Such photographs were often used in photo albums and as gifts. They were so inexpensive that most people had the means to purchase them.[30] Photographs of the deceased were also produced in calling-card format such as the one in figure 44, especially head-and-shoulders shots and full-length shots of the deceased and the coffin. Photographs in larger formats were more expensive. The "parlor photograph" (*kabinettfotografi*) was about 4 × 6 inches (11 × 16 cm) in size.[31] Figure 45 is an intermediate format, between the calling card and parlor photograph in size. The actual photograph, which is small, is mounted on a large cardboard mat, which indicates that it was meant to be framed.

The replies to the Nordic Museum's questionnaire on photography contain a considerable amount of information about the uses of portrait photography in Sweden around the turn of the twentieth century. According to the informants, photographs were often taken in connection with important events (or rites of passage) such as confirmations, military service, school graduations, marriage engagements, and weddings. Other events mentioned included day trips and more extensive travels, visits to county fairs, general holiday celebrations, and gatherings of family and friends prior to someone leaving for America. When traveling photographers came to visit, they took pictures of homes and farms. Calling cards were often purchased by the dozen and put in albums, exchanged between friends and family, or sent to relatives in America. Photographs were often kept in a dresser drawer and taken out when guests visited. They might also be kept in a bowl. Large-format pictures might be tacked to the wall or displayed in frames.[32] People used photographs of deceased persons in the same ways they used other photographs. The breakup of family units that came with increased mobility in the era of urbanization and emigration made such photographs popular. Those who could not participate in a funeral could still have a memory of it.

In a study based on thirteen private photo collections from Denmark, Norway, and Iceland, Danish scholar Johanne Maria Jensen has shown that portrait photographs of the deceased were put in family albums and hung on walls.[33] She found examples of photographs of the deceased from as early as the 1840s, the first decade of photography. Following the introduction of less expensive and simpler methods of photographic reproduction in the 1860s, which made it possible to produce many paper prints from the same negative, the genre became increasingly common. Jensen found that death was in fact one of the first subjects people chose to commemorate in their personal photo collections. In the earliest days of photography, people did not associate the new technology with special events, so the custom of photographing the deceased became established before the photographing of weddings, engagements, confirmations, christenings, and similar events.

It is difficult to determine how people regarded these photographs and what significance they placed on them. Jensen points out an important context: the deceased were kept in the home until the funeral, were neatly dressed and groomed, and were viewed by funeral guests. Because of this, most people were accustomed to the sight of a dead person. Although death could be just as frightening and distressing in those days as it is now, it held a visual place in culture and in people's consciousness. The photographs did not portray disease, painful moments of death, or heart-rending grief but instead were peaceful, beautiful representations of death. If these pictures appear frightening or macabre to modern-day observers, it is partly because we are no longer accustomed to seeing corpses close up. The private photographs of the deceased are also markedly different from the dramatic depictions of the dead in the mass media, where unknown bodies are often used to gain readers' attention.[34]

A Critical Voice from the Archives

One of the informants who answered the questionnaire on portrait photography expressed a strongly negative opinion of photographs of the deceased. Her reply is comparatively long. She was born in 1889 in the town of Skurup in the province of Skåne. According to her, photographing a corpse lying in its coffin was common in the 1890s and a few years into the 1900s. Such photographs were especially popular when no portrait of the person had been taken during his or her lifetime. The informant did not like this photographic practice:

> People have even framed these pictures and hung them on the walls, and given them away to relatives and friends, where they are mixed together with other pictures in albums and bowls of photos. Terrible![35]

She maintained that opinions were sharply divided regarding the aptness of photographing corpses. She also made the point that taking a portrait photograph after death might be disrespectful and might go against the wishes of the deceased; a dead person could not protest, even if the individual had been opposed to having his or her picture taken during life.[36] The informant was particularly critical of a farm family to whom she was related. In the 1890s they commissioned a photograph of a deceased three-year-old boy who had died of a contagious childhood disease. The dead boy was dressed up in a suit he had never been able to wear while alive and was propped up in a chair to be photographed.

> This parlor-sized photo was put behind glass and framed, and hung on the wall among their framed lithographs. They were happy to have a photograph of

him that looked as though he were alive. The only thing you noticed was the somewhat loose way he held his body and the vague look of the eyes. Later on, sometime between 1905–15, when the traveling agents from the photo enlargement companies were going through the countryside, this photo was enlarged. This pleased those to whom the boy had belonged, but in the opinion of me and many others, it was very repulsive from beginning to end.[37]

The photograph mentioned here was thus of the type that according to Jay Ruby was common in the United States, in which the corpse was depicted as though it were alive. However, I have found no such portraits in Swedish photography archives.

To what did the critical voices object? Why did they dislike the custom of photographing deceased persons? There have been many different opinions about practice since the end of the nineteenth century. Many went to considerable expense and effort to have deceased relatives photographed; others found the practice distasteful. It became clear that during the first half of the twentieth century seeing the deceased in photographs was offensive to the sensibilities of many. Whether this is a modern attitude per se is difficult to say. It may be connected to the fact that people became less accustomed to seeing dead bodies as the custom of keeping the deceased in the home until the funeral fell out of practice and the custom of viewing the dead body slowly diminished.

Despite the modernity of photography and the long-standing tradition of death portraits, this photographic genre did not survive in modern visual culture. While death disappeared from family photo albums, new types of photographs became more frequent. At the end of the twentieth century, people happily photographed an event that would have been unimaginable one hundred years earlier: the beginning of life. A century earlier, photographs of pregnant bellies, nursing babies, and the moment of delivery were as nonexistent in private photo albums as death is today.[38]

If the modern technology of photography could capture death and make the dead eternally present, another modern technology was focused instead on obliterating the corpse. Chapter 6 will deal with the introduction and establishment of cremation as a modern alternative to burial.

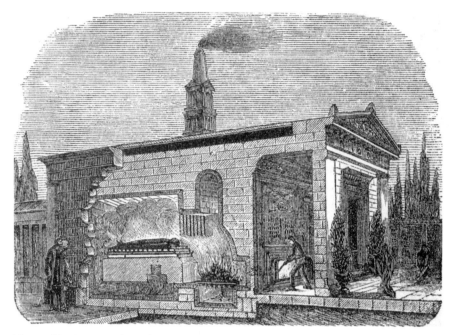

Figure 46. Crematorium shown in cross-section, complete with burning corpse, a fireman, and smoke pouring from the chimney. Like those who view this illustration, the observer standing to the left seems to be able to see through the building's walls. From Per Lindell, *Likbränningen jemte öfriga grafskick* (Stockholm, 1888), 407. Duplication: Kungl. biblioteket - National Library of Sweden.

Chapter Six

Purifying Flames

No, never let me be buried,
when my earthly journey's through.
My body I cannot and will not give
to feed the worms of the soil,
no, purified by fire, may it rise,
like my soul, to the heavens!

—Ernst Arendorff

A crematorium furnace, or incinerator, produces temperatures of up to 1,000 degrees Celsius (ca. 1,800 degrees Fahrenheit). The extremely hot air burns a body in just over one hour without exposing it to open flames. The first crematorium in Sweden was erected in Stockholm in 1887 through the efforts of the Swedish Cremation Society (Svenska Likbränningsföreningen), but this new technology did not begin to gain general acceptance until the 1930s. In the beginning, it was primarily Sweden's urban, middle-class elite who supported what they saw as a modern, hygienic, and aesthetically appealing way of handling dead human bodies. The basic impetus for the cremation movement was the perception that earth burial was repulsive. The idea of the body being eaten by microorganisms and worms was so repugnant to some people that they were prepared to invest considerable energy in solving the technical, political, financial, and cultural problems that stood in the way of "the funeral practice of the future."[1]

During the late eighteenth and early nineteenth centuries, the problem of how to deal with dead human bodies became increasingly difficult. Large cities on the European continent began to replace their crowded, smelly inner-city burial grounds with park-like cemeteries on the municipal outskirts. The Cimétière de Père Lachaise in Paris, established in 1804, became a model for many new cemeteries. The family graves of the bourgeoisie were expensive monuments erected in exclusive, landscaped settings, while those who could not afford funerary extravagance were buried at the outer edges of the cemetery or in other, simpler cemeteries. In this way, the new cemeteries of the nineteenth century reflected

the contemporary class structure of society. In Sweden, the Norra Kyrkogården cemetery opened in Solna, just outside Stockholm's city limits, in
1827. It was laid out according to a formal park plan, with symmetrical
quarters divided by paths. The cemetery was planted with many trees, not
only for the sake of beauty but also because trees were believed to purify
the earth and air from poisons that caused disease.[2]

Human bodies and their disposal were defined as a hygienic and aesthetic problem with which national and city governments had to come to
terms. A number of solutions were suggested. As early as the late eighteenth century, the old custom of burying church and government officials inside churches ended.[3] The smell was troublesome, especially in the
warm summer months, and the corpses were believed to infect the living
with disease by means of miasmatic evaporation through the church floor.
In bringing church entombments to an end, lawmakers solved both the
aesthetic and hygienic aspects of the problem in one step. Church burial
was a centuries-old practice, and corpses must have smelled long before
the end of the eighteenth century. In earlier times, though, having tombs
within church walls, close to the altar and the saints, was considered more
important than the discomfort offensive odors caused the living. The smell
was not considered a problem, which indicates that sensitivity to odors is a
culturally determined and historically specific phenomenon. But from the
late eighteenth century onward, disintegrating corpses were increasingly
perceived as poisonous and upsetting.

As the population of Swedish cities increased along with the industrialization of the late nineteenth century, so did the interest in creating healthier city environments. This included considerations of how to reduce the
potential dangers decaying corpses posed to the living. Dead bodies came to
be regarded as refuse (albeit of a special sort) that should be handled effi-
ciently, just like garbage, slaughterhouse offal, and sewage. The new science
of bacteriology brought deeper understanding of contagion and influenced
discussions of how to handle dead bodies.[4] Corpses became a concern for
city planners and public health officials. In cities and later in the countryside as well, corpse sheds and mortuaries were constructed so people no
longer had to keep the deceased in the home. The proper drainage of cemetery land became a priority, and rules were established as to how soon a
grave plot could be reused and the depth at which coffins had to be buried.
Urbanization, new means of transport (trains, steamboats, automobiles),
and the population's increased mobility also led to increased traffic of dead
bodies, which called for more regulations.

Cremation was an effective way of rendering corpses harmless and easy to
handle: sterile, compact, odorless, lightweight. But cremation is about more
than rationality. Its symbolic meanings were just as important, as this chapter describes.

Purity

Cremation advocates frequently used "purity" as a theme in their writings, which often had a hygienic theme, especially in the first decades after the establishment of the Swedish Cremation Society in 1882.[5] Purity was also significant on a symbolic level.

The Hygienic Argument

When cremationists advocated their cause, the argument they used most frequently was that cremation was greatly preferable to interment from a hygienic point of view. Even when not writing specifically about hygiene, they usually made reference to the purity or cleanliness of cremation. The enthusiastic advocates presented cremation's hygienic aspects as indisputable, which gave them an air of scientific authority combined with progressive social activism. Many members of the Swedish Cremation Society were doctors or were employed in other fields involving hygiene issues. Stockholm's surgeon general, Klas Linroth, for instance, was engaged in all matters of hygiene and was one of the driving forces of the Swedish Cremation Society from its inception.

Curt Wallis, a professor of pathology who later became a member of the board of directors of the Swedish Cremation Society, wrote an article published in *Hygiea* at the early date of 1877. The article is written in a strict and rational scientific style. Wallis's intention was more to examine and report on the benefits of cremation than to actually advocate its introduction. However, this style of argumentation became widely used among the cremationists. Wallis addressed his medical colleagues when he wrote:

> Because of the practical spirit of our time, we are led to regard the matter [of burial] primarily from the viewpoint of the care of public health, as being the most important [issue]. Do the bodies of the deceased, cared for in the method now in use, and which has been in general use for many centuries, comprise a true danger to the health of the living? And if, by an improvement in this [traditional] method, we were not able to avoid these dangers, and yet by the introduction of cremation were able to avoid them, then the question will already have been decided to the advantage of cremation, if in fact the living place a value upon their health, upon which point there can be no doubt. To decide this matter, it will be necessary to delve into several details concerning the chemical processes which the bodies of the dead undergo once life has left the body.[6]

A long and detailed description of what happens to bodies buried in various types of ground follows—for example, if the soil is wet, bodies putrefy and rot rather than decompose. Wallis concludes that

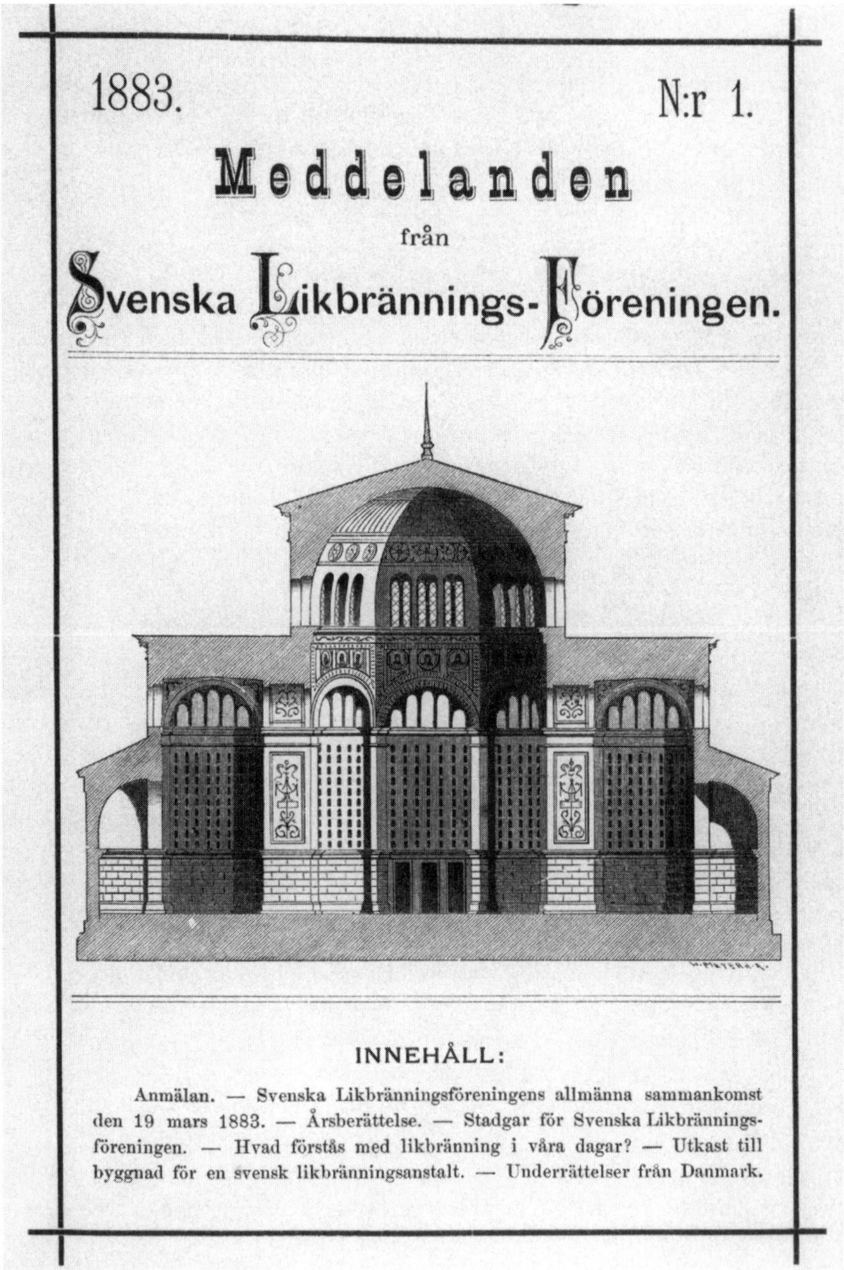

1883.   N:r 1.

Meddelanden

från

Svenska Likbrännings-Föreningen.

INNEHÅLL:

Anmälan. — Svenska Likbränningsföreningens allmänna sammankomst den 19 mars 1883. — Årsberättelse. — Stadgar för Svenska Likbrännings-föreningen. — Hvad förstås med likbränning i våra dagar? — Utkast till byggnad för en svensk likbränningsanstalt. — Underrättelser från Danmark.

Figure 47. The cover of the first issue of *Meddelanden från Svenska Librännningsföreningen* (1883). Duplication: Kungl. biblioteket - National Library of Sweden.

in the most favorable case, burial provides the same results [as cremation], i.e., the complete disintegration of the body, but [it] can never with full certainty preclude the possibility of a much less favorable result, consisting of the introduction of the products of putrefaction into the water which seeps from cemeteries. Just as certainly as we prefer certainty over great likelihood in the fulfillment of our wishes, we should also prefer cremation before burial from the standpoint of hygiene.[7]

In an 1884 article in the periodical *Meddelanden från Svenska Likbränningsföreningen* (*Announcements from the Swedish Cremation Society*), physician and later national medical adviser Richard Wawrinsky also criticized earth burial from a "sanitary standpoint." He maintained that dead bodies produced poisons, and he encouraged changes in the ways corpses were stored and handled. In addition, he had opinions regarding the types of materials that should be used in caskets and grave clothes, as well as where cemeteries should be located. The most hygienic solution, according to Wawrinsky, was to adopt the cremation of dead bodies.[8]

Per Lindell was an engineer, a writer, and the strongest voice and initiator of the Swedish Cremation Society. He based his 1888 book *Likbränningen jemte öfriga grafskick* (*Cremation and Other Funerary Practices*) on a number of medical, scientific, and scholarly sources from Sweden and abroad. The book is 434 pages long and contains many illustrations and tables. Since it deals mostly with the disadvantages of other funeral practices and the advantages of cremation, it is basically propaganda for the cremationist cause.

Most articles dealing with cremation from the standpoint of hygiene follow a certain pattern. The articles often begin with the demand that the method by which we choose to bury our dead should present no risks to the living. This is followed by an account of the dangers of traditional earth burial and the difficulty of establishing cemeteries that offer satisfactory conditions. Finally, the articles state that with regard to cleanliness and health, no funeral practice can compete with cremation. The hygiene arguments are also often combined with other arguments of a practical nature. For example, urns require less room than caskets and thus offer a way to check the rapid expansion of cemeteries as a result of increased population and migration to urban areas. Cremation is also less expensive, both for society and the individual.

Wallis's text, quoted earlier, and the articles on the hygienic aspects of burial published in *Meddelanden* during the 1880s contain statements that show that knowledge of bacteriology and contagion was not especially well developed. In rather vague terms, the authors wrote about "the products of decay," "health-threatening gases," and "poisonous compounds" that could be disseminated into the air and water. Pathogenic, disease-causing bacteria were not mentioned until 1900, in an article by F. Levison (chair of the

Danish Society for Cremation). This coincided with a rather late general acceptance of bacteriology in Sweden (Robert Koch had proved the germ theory of disease back in the early 1880s).[9] In his article, Levison carefully reviewed "definitely stated" research results regarding the capacity of different types of bacteria to survive and spread in soil. He concluded that cremation was healthier than burial. Like many others in *Meddelanden*, this article is fairly long-winded in its presentation of numbers and research results.[10] The use of statistics and science to strengthen an argument was a widespread rhetorical tactic in turn-of-the-twentieth-century culture; the cremation movement used it to signal modernity and scientific substance.[11]

Thus, around 1900 the most common arguments for the adoption of cremation were its hygienic advantages. Public health was a current topic, and the general public was ready to accept this type of argument. In social and political contexts as well as scientific ones, questions of health and hygiene were frequently discussed. Opponents of cremation found it difficult to rebut the sanitary issues. Cremation stood out as the healthy funeral practice for the modern age. Interest in hygiene had started to blossom in the 1870s and had only grown stronger. Numerous writings were published on the subject from the perspectives of both conventional and alternative medicine. Using words of honor such as "purity" and "natural," writers advocated various health teachings with partially religious or utopian content.[12]

When Sweden's new law on health care was adopted in 1874, cities were required to establish boards of health. Scientific experts were thus charged with keeping watch over hygiene and cleanliness issues. Interest in these questions also resulted in scientific research on health care. During this period of intense industrialization, matters of hygiene reached a breakthrough: urbanization, new ways of living and working, and greater social and geographic mobility affected people's health and created demands for social action.[13] Viewed against this background, the engagement of so many doctors in the Swedish Cremation Society emerges as typical for the time.

In the beginning of the twentieth century, arguments about hygiene and sanitation became less important in the cremationist rhetoric. Writings from this period refer to hygiene in an offhand way and without further explanation or embellishment. This does not necessarily mean that hygiene had ceased to be a viable argument. As Swedish ethnographers Jonas Frykman and Orvar Löfgren have pointed out, hygiene was still "the great keyword of the Interwar years." The word occurred in many combinations, such as *skolhygien* (school hygiene), *samhällshygien* (social hygiene), *arvshygien* (hereditary hygiene), and even *väghygien* (road hygiene).[14] By the interwar years, the word "hygiene" was extremely well established. Simply using this word allowed the cremation movement to point out the modernity of its cause and its place within a larger context of social renewal.

In the Swedish context, the case for cremation was pursued not by the state or municipalities but by private individuals organized into an association. Although cremation societies were formed in countries throughout the Western world, in other countries the development moved in different directions. In some cases, crematoriums were built and managed by these societies; in other cases they were built by private cemetery owners or wealthy donors; in still other places, crematoriums were administered by churches or municipal governments.[15] In Sweden, a mixed model developed: in the beginning, crematoriums were owned by the Swedish Cremation Society, but eventually they came to be owned and managed by the Church of Sweden or the respective municipalities.[16]

The Aesthetic Argument

Cleanliness and purity were central values touted by the advocates of cremation, and not only in the hygienic sense. The concept of purity was also applied to cremation as a process and to its final result. Burning human remains was viewed as a process of purification. The body was purified by fire, and the final product was a clean, harmless substance. In cremationist rhetoric, two contrasting images were often played against one another: on one hand, the repulsive, horrible process of decay that took place in the grave and, on the other, the purifying burning process, which left a clean white ash.[17] The seemingly rational hygienic arguments for cremation are thus interwoven with a romantic symbolism of purity.

The symbolic value of purity also characterized what cremationists pointed out as the "aesthetic" advantages of the new funeral practice over earth burial. Burial was interpreted as ugly and dirty, while cremation was seen as beautiful and clean. This new, appealing funeral practice would also bring about a new view of death: through the symbolism of cremation, the despair, horror, and darkness associated with death would be replaced by lighter, more beautiful thoughts. This resembles the hygienic argument: since the old method injures living humans, it should be replaced with something new. However, the aesthetic argument has more to do with how people's emotions are affected by experiences connected with the grave and thoughts of what happens "down there." As Belgian symbolist writer Maurice Maeterlinck, frequently quoted in publications of the Swedish cremation movement, expressed it: "Decay offends our senses, stains our memory, slays our courage. But purified by fire, the memory lives on in the ether as a glorious idea, and death is nothing more than undying birth in a cradle of flame."[18]

Proclamations of cremation's aesthetic superiority occur throughout the period, connected with the idea that prevailing perceptions of death were unnecessarily or even injuriously dismal—a fact that would be rectified by the

introduction of cremation. The aesthetic dimension of cremation supposedly included an ethical and even a socio-psychological aspect: the adoption
of cremation would generate a healthier relationship with death. Cremation
had the capacity to bring a "lighter view of the mystery of death."[19]

This idea was expressed strongly in 1927 by cremation enthusiast Ingeborg Olson. According to Olson, death had become a ghost that haunted
her contemporaries, a ghost that threatened "to halt the dance, silence
the music, end the eager work, stop the clock, just when all has reached its
best tempo."[20] For Olson, the funeral practices, not death itself, were the
problem:

> Burial in the ground has created around itself such an atmosphere of dis-
> consolation and darkness, of cold and horror, which has planted itself in our
> thoughts, ideas and associations, colored our entire imagination, our realm of
> thought, our attitude to life, the world and death, and has been passed down
> from generation to generation.[21]

The custom of earth burial gave rise to superstition, fear, and terror. It was
always somber, but it was especially ill suited for modern humans, for it
had become "a greater contradiction than previously." According to Olson,
human beings were inflicted with the fear of death as children by being
present at funerals. She felt children should be spared from "standing at
the black pit, where we face that threatening, unknown something called
Death." Instead, children should "learn to know the dissolution of the dead
body by fire," which would create a strongly different impression so that
death would lose its terror, if not its sting.

Thus the majesty of death would prevail among humans, rather than
the terrifying ghost that "we must push into the innermost corners of
our consciousness in order to forget."[22] Olson felt the dignity and purity
of cremation would reform funeral practices in general. It would bring
simplicity and equality in the face of death by abolishing the tradition of
elaborate grave monuments. It would also end the barbaric and objec-
tionable custom of comforting oneself with food and drink at the wake
after the horrible experience in the cemetery. She regarded the custom
of the funeral feast as an "offensive cult of death." Olson felt that after
the beautiful experience cremation presented, no artificial consolation
would be needed.

> If one goes home with the sure knowledge that the dissolution of the body,
> which in the earth takes years and years, is now already complete; that the
> dear departed one is a handful of dust upon the sea of eternity, then one's
> thoughts—freed from concerns about the dead body and the horrible pro-
> cess to which it is exposed in the ground—may fly to the only true effects left
> behind by the deceased: his or her memory.[23]

Cremation Poetry

The Swedish Cremation Society's journal, *Meddelanden,* often published poetry on the theme of purifying flames. Sometimes there were quotations from ancient Greek and Roman poems, sometimes excerpted parts of hymns or other texts that originally had nothing to do with cremation but that happened to contain one or more lines about ashes, death, or fire. The most frequently quoted "cremation poem" in Sweden was "Bön vid lågorna" ("A Prayer before the Flames") by the celebrated poet Verner von Heidenstam. Heidenstam was a member of the Cremation Society and sometimes allowed his name to be used as a drawing card, for example, at the 1923 Gothenburg Exposition. The Cremation Society had a pavilion there, with an outdoor columbarium and chapel. Gustav Schlyter, one of the society members who arranged the project, saw to it that Heidenstam was made honorary chair of the exposition's organizing committee.[24] Heidenstam's poem was published occasionally in *Meddelanden,* sometimes under the heading "Statements about Cremation," among other quotations from famous and not-so-famous persons. The poem is characterized less by the idea of purity than by a mysticism of fire, in which the flames free the spirit from the body:

> Holy Spirit, thee I pray.
> Fire and vict'ry song Thy name,
> spirit of trial and tribulation,
> a light o'er tears and death forlorn,
> burn to ash our human form!
> In Thy eternal flames I place
> from death, in prayer, my embrace.[25]

Here, fire is a holy spirit. Other cremation poems present a more traditional Christian view, combined with the idea of the purification of the body by fire, as in the poem "Resurrection," signed simply by "Gret."

> My remains, which are burned to ash,
> shall one day rise again.
> Human, by the name you're known,
> shall your Jesus call you then.
> The body, cleans'ed by the flames,
> the soul, fallen in its battle
> against the sin of all the earth, is united
> with a Spirit, good and mild.[26]

Still other poems are more explicit and propagandistic. Earth burial is contrasted with cremation. The poet makes a concise statement about a subject to which the more scientifically oriented cremationists devoted many detail-filled pages: what happens to the dead body in the grave is unhealthy, while flames, on the other hand, purify it.

> My body shall the worms of decay ne'er touch—
> No, pure flame alone shall consume it!
> I loved the light, which all things warms,
> and therefore I burn; lay me not in the grave![27]

Implicit in this idea of purification by fire is a conception of the dead body as something filthy that must be cleansed. Much more could be said about these poems (and there are many more in the cremationists' publications), but here it is sufficient to see them as a unique element in the cremation movement's rhetoric about the capacity of fire to purify the body.[28]

The cremation movement's campaign to make perceptions of death lighter and more beautiful also included a creative relationship with the Swedish language. The coining of a more appealing set of idioms was an important part of the aesthetic program. In Swedish, the word first used for cremation was *likbränning*, literally "corpse burning." In the long run, this term was too explicit to satisfy the cremationists' aesthetic preferences. It was replaced by a peculiar new word perceived as more suitable: *eldbegängelse* ("committal by fire"). The word was constructed in 1887 by Henrik Hedlund, a cremation advocate and editor of the major newspaper *Göteborgs Handels- och Sjöfartstidning*. Oscar Övden wrote in his history of the cremation movement in Sweden, *Eldbegängelsens historia i Sverige 1882–1932*, that this word was a translation of the German *Feuerbestattung*, "invented" by Professor Karl Reclam of Leipzig.[29] The original name of the Swedish Cremation Society, Svenska Likbrännings-föreningen, was based on the older term. In 1918 the society changed its name to the more aesthetically pleasing Svenska Edlbegängelseföreningen. Övden himself consistently used more "beautiful" idioms, such as *stoft* ("dust" or "remains") instead of *lik* ("corpse"), and the somewhat contrived verb *eldbegå* ("to commit by fire"). In his overview of the language employed by the cremation movement, Övden expressed joy over the beautiful new words. For example, he found the Latin-based *incinerator* more suitable than the Swedish *ugn* (literally "oven" or "furnace"), "that unappealing word . . . which gives an altogether faulty idea of cremation."[30] For Övden, language usage was an important element in the cremationist program:

> Developments have provided the cremationists with a number of beautiful words; these must not be lost. They are an achievement, and for many, are just as valuable as the technological ones by which cremation is so beautifully carried out.[31]

Eventually, the word *eldbegängelse* was forsaken for the term *kremering* ("cremation"), *eldbegängelsetempel* for *krematorium*, and so on.[32] The poetic qualities of

Övden's favorite words were replaced by more technical and neutral terms. The development of Swedish cremation terminology proceeded hand in hand with the development of the cremation movement itself: the romantic and ideological elements were eventually neutralized, especially in the years following World War II.

Spaces and Rituals

Swedish crematoriums were designed in accordance with the concepts of purity, light, and symbolism of fire. As early as 1964, art historian Ulf G. Johnsson stated in the art history journal *Konsthistorisk tidskrift* that crematorium buildings were interesting objects for research: they offered "a rather unique opportunity to study how an ideology seeks aesthetic expressions and how these are realized architecturally."[33] According to Johnsson, the design of the first European crematoriums, inspired by classical architecture, set the standards.

In addition to the various practical/technical spaces and installations, such as an autopsy room, corpse storage, casket receiving area, incinerator, and chimney, a crematorium must also house a room for rituals. Attempts were made to hide all practical elements through ingenious architecture. For example, at the Helsingborg Crematorium the chimney was disguised to look like a column topped by a gold sculpture.[34] Johnsson also reflected on the duality within the rhetoric of cremation advocates, with "hygienic/practical" arguments on the one hand and "ethical/aesthetic" arguments on the other.[35] To me, these two arguments are aspects of the same issue or conceptual complex, expressed in different ways.

The (ideal) design for crematoriums, especially the ceremonial rooms, was a topic of discussion within cremationist circles. Gustav Schlyter developed his own religious/Romantic program, which found concrete expression in the Baltiska Templet (Baltic Temple), the Swedish Cremation Society's exhibition building at the 1914 Baltic Exposition in Malmö.[36] The proponents of cremation deemed the ritual functions and meanings of the spaces to have significant or even central importance. The effort to convince the public, the authorities, and the church to accept the new funeral custom was one reason so much attention was devoted to architecture and rituals. But the cremation movement itself also contained many disparate ideological elements that its members wanted to make manifest.[37]

The ways cremation was actually practiced varied from country to country. In Sweden, for example, it has never been common to spread cremated ashes to the wind. Sweden also has relatively strict laws regarding what can be done with the ashes. In Great Britain, however, it has been common since cremation was first employed to spread cremated ashes. At the first English crematorium in Golders Green, a large lawn was laid out for this purpose.[38] Cremationists were free to design the entire process as they desired, from the rituals to the actual cremation to the disposal of the ashes. The first crematorium on the European continent, built in Milan in 1876, had no ceremonial room. The building was almost entirely filled with urn niches, and the incinerator was set up in a relatively small room, where gurneys could be pulled directly from the storage room to the incinerator doors. In Sweden, crematoriums were designed to look like chapels, and at first the committal ceremony imitated that of earth burial, so that the casket was lowered and disappeared at the end of the ceremony.[39] Many cremationists criticized this approach. Some preferred that the casket be conveyed away horizontally instead, and a number of crematoriums were built according to this idea.[40] Eventually a third approach became the Swedish model: the casket remains in place until the funeral party has left the room.[41]

It is interesting that it was taken for granted that the practice of cremation should contain a ritual element. Other possibilities are conceivable: both Christian and anti-church cremationists could have made arguments for not surrounding cremation with rituals. Crematoriums could have been simple, functional facilities for the handling of corpses. This was not the case, however, which indicates that cremation was not merely a practical, rational issue. The cultural and emotional aspects were more important to the successful introduction of cremation. The new fear and sensitivity toward what happened to a corpse buried in a grave called for a reform that could respond to these fears. That response was cremation. To be successfully introduced to Sweden, cremation needed concrete forms and expressions.

The crematorium facilities built in the concentration camps of Nazi Germany had a completely different character. No importance was placed on handling the deceased with care and piety or on seeing to it that they were given a ceremonial farewell. Rather, the purpose of those facilities was to dispose of large numbers of dead bodies using the lowest possible fuel expenditure. No attempt was made to conceal the chimneys in the architecture, and the incinerators were designed with two or three parallel chambers that could all be operated simultaneously. In Auschwitz, there were fifty-two fixed incineration chambers and two mobile ones. Several bodies could be incinerated in one chamber at once, and no caskets were used.[42]

For the sake of comparing their design with Swedish crematoriums, I will set aside the terrible role these crematoriums played in facilitating the Holocaust. Swedish cremation advocates claimed that the meaning of cremation could be found in its rational nature, and they tried to convince the public of its advantages through reason. If it were a simple matter of disposing of dead human bodies effectively, they could have built crematoriums like the ones in Auschwitz. But the cremation movement wanted to transform the ritual aspects of death rather than discard them. For this reason, reverence and beauty were central values. In a Swedish crematorium, the incinerators, cold storage rooms, and other technical spaces are not open to funeral participants and can only be reached through a back entrance. The technology must provide service without being seen. But the ritual room is given primary importance: it is artfully decorated and placed centrally, with a grand entrance and a lobby.[43]

It is remarkable that knowledge of the Holocaust crematoriums does not appear to have influenced people's attitudes toward cremation in the years following World War II. Despite the fact that the Nazis' diabolical cremation machinery was used to eliminate their victims, cremation became increasingly common in Sweden, the United Kingdom, and other non-Catholic Western countries.[44] This indicates that the funeral ceremonies of peacetime cremation, and the respectful handling of the remains of the dead associated with it, have set it apart from the industrial horror of the concentration camps. Expressed another way, the technological similarities between these two ways of handling the dead are perceived as less prominent than the symbolic, cultural differences between them.[45]

Technology

The first crematorium incinerators were constructed in the 1870s. Cremation activists regarded them as a decisive factor for the successful introduction of cremation to Sweden. In a 1925 article on cremation technology, Gustav Schlyter wrote:

> Today, the modern cremation movement may look back upon fifty years of service. This is due to the solution, just a half a century ago, of the technological problems: the construction of an incineration apparatus which possessed characteristics which would allow it to be approved for the dissolution of dead human bodies.[46]

What characteristics were required of an incinerator? First, cremation had to be clean and efficient. The "dissolution" of the dead body needed to proceed as smoothly as possible. Burning a human body on a bonfire, as practiced in Scandinavia in ancient times and in India, was not an option in the modern Western world (although bodies had been burned on open fires several times during the nineteenth century, in Europe as well as North America).[47] The problem needed a technological solution, in accordance with the concept of the new funeral practice as "pure." Schlyter's article describes a new cremator unit from the Höganäs Corporation, outlining what was required of the technology:

Undeniably, a prerequisite for the concept of cremation to gain acceptance is that the incineration process itself can be achieved in a religiously and aesthetically appealing manner. In addition, because crematoria must be built in or near cities, there is the definite need

- that the incineration can be carried out quickly,
- that it shall proceed securely and completely, and not leave half-incinerated or charred remains,
- that the incineration will take place only in a furnace which is used exclusively for this purpose,
- that the incineration does not create smoke or offensive-smelling gases,
- that the ash will be clean and white, and that it can be collected quickly and conveniently,
- that the furnace as well as the incineration be inexpensive, and
- that numerous incinerations may be conducted immediately one after the other.[48]

In ways both practical and symbolic, the design of crematorium incinerators thus embodied an entire ideology of death. The technical solutions were derived from industrial incineration technology. However, specific requirements were placed on this particular application of the technology, since the task at hand was burning human bodies, which had to be treated with special respect even if they could be regarded as a type of refuse.

The demands of speed, efficiency, and cleanliness are derived from the cremationists' critique of earth burial as slow, inefficient, and dirty. They are also tied to the honored principles of aesthetics and reverence. Yet speed, efficiency, and cleanliness are also values in their own right. The cremationists wanted to create a *modern* method of handling the dead body: the dead could be burned with industrial efficiency in a production line setting; it was inexpensive; it was quick, clean, and odor-free, and it left behind no unpleasant by-products. If technology can symbolize efficiency and modernity, incinerator technology is a symbol of the cremationists' values and efforts.

Architectural or engineering-type drawings of incinerator designs were frequently used as illustrations in the Cremation Society's journal. For those without a background in engineering, these drawings can be difficult to comprehend. Although a significant number of the society's members were engineers, most were not, and drawings such as the one in figure 49 were not purely informational—they signaled expert knowledge, efficiency, and modernity.

A new genre of technical drawings was created by and for engineers during the nineteenth century. By 1870, an identifiable pictorial language was established in engineering journals and textbooks that included illustrations.

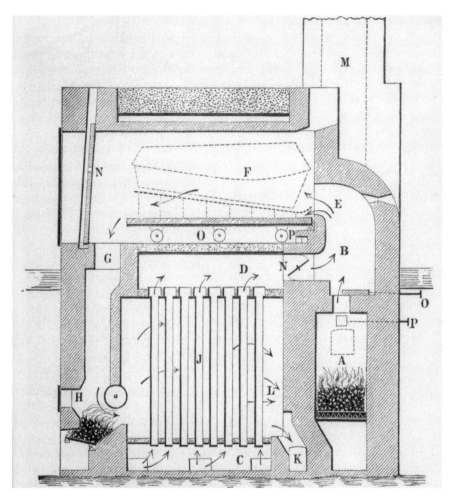

Figure 48. "A cross-section of the apparatus," that is, the cremation furnace Colonel Klingenstierna constructed in 1887 for the first crematorium in Sweden. From Per Lindell, *Likbränningen jemte öfriga grafskick* (Stockholm, 1888), 412. Duplication: Kungl. biblioteket - National Library of Sweden.

The pictures became increasingly professional and standardized and were usually designed in the form of architectural drawings or schematics. The illustrations communicated nonverbally. Earlier, these illustrations had been more straightforward and easy for laypeople to understand (compare figure 46). During the period 1800–1870, the illustrations increasingly focused on details while also becoming more abstract, with charts and cross-section views. At the same time, improved printing methods allowed publishers to reproduce drawings in greater detail.[49] They were thus more indirectly important in creating a readiness among the middle class to embrace and support technology and technological applications in industry and society; members of this social group viewed themselves as modern and became a "technology-bearing stratum."[50] By utilizing the visual culture of engineers, the Swedish Cremation Society demonstrated its membership in, and turned its attentions toward, the technology-bearing stratum of the day.

A notable characteristic of the cremation movement in its early years was a belief in progress and technology.[51] Some of the writers in *Meddelanden* conveyed a particularly strong enthusiasm for the benefits of technology. To them, the very possibility of constructing efficient crematoriums would have been reason enough for the public to accept the new funeral technique. An article from 1883 bursts with excitement over the possibilities offered by technology:

> Placed in the retort chamber, the dead body is quickly and easily transformed, without releasing any dangerous or ill-smelling gases into the open air. For a corpse in the grave, the process of transformation takes about 20 years, more or less, depending upon the type of soil and the agents used to delay the decay. By contrast, in the cremation facilities built thus far, this entire process takes about 1½ hours, which likely could be shortened to approximately 30 minutes, or about the same amount of time needed to fill in a grave after the casket has been lowered into it. The incineration itself may be achieved in one of two ways: either with or without flames. In the latter case, the chamber is filled with air heated to one or several thousand degrees [Celsius], which flows around the corpse in a consuming stream. Both burn methods provide the same result. They transform all organic substances in the human body into gaseous form, leaving only the inorganic, unburnable components, the so-called bone dust or ash. This method not only prevents the creation of the actual products of decay which occur in the grave, and the pests associated with them, including worms, but also completely destroys all of the dangerous substances which are often contained in a dead body as the result of contagious disease, and which are spread by its natural disintegration, in some cases many years after burial. The ash, or bone dust, which remains after incineration is completely clean and white.[52]

A number of the statements here are identical to those in the Höganäs Corporation's description of its furnace cited earlier. Nonetheless, forty-two years had passed between the publications of the two texts.[53] There is a striking consistency in the presentations of cremation technology: references to its efficiency, cleanliness, and harmlessness occur again and again. It is also interesting that ideas of purity are associated with the ash, which is "clean and white." White, the color of innocence and purity, provides a symbolic guarantee that the technology works. No other results, such as brown or grayish-black remains, would have been satisfactory. What is left unmentioned is that when the "ash" is removed from the incinerator, it almost always contains large pieces of bone that must be ground up to ensure that the remains have a fine consistency and can be perceived as ash.

Interestingly, the same attitudes recur in a Swedish company's presentation of its incinerators in a brochure from the 1980s. In English, the company claims that its product satisfies the need for "efficient cremation under hygienic conditions with smokeless operation." The system guarantees "smoke- odor- and dustless operation." In addition, the system is said to be forward-looking and to combine experience with modern innovation.[54]

The requirement that the technology used in cremation allow for odorless and smoke-free incineration is thus over one hundred years old. From the start, the cremation movement wanted the cremation process to be invisible from the outside. The ideal was to hide the process of destroying corpses by burning them.[55] The architecture of crematoriums contributed by making the technology invisible to visitors.[56]

Another theme emerges from these texts: smoke and odor do in fact occur during cremation, and this is perceived as problematic. The marketing presentations of cremation technology from the 1980s claim that the gases released would *normally* be rendered smoke- and odor-free. One hundred years after the construction of the first Swedish crematorium furnace, achieving this was still technically difficult. Making the chimney invisible and eliminating the more noticeable traces of cremation is, I would argue, a component of the cremation movement's "aesthetic" strivings. The new funeral technique allowed for dead bodies to disappear almost magically, thanks to ingenious machinery. All that came out of the incinerator was clean, white ash, which was supposed to eradicate the thought of rotting corpses. But it was equally important to prevent people from imagining what went on inside an incinerator.

Cremation and Modernity

The development of cremation is intertwined with the emergence of modern society. The problems cremationists sought to solve originated in a specific historical context. Today, the dead body is associated with other problems. Both earth burial and cremation are harmful to the environment, releasing substances such as mercury into the soil and water. Cremation also uses large amounts of energy, and in Sweden attempts have been made to recycle the heat from crematoriums. A contemporary movement demands environmentally friendly, or "green," funerals (especially in Britain). In Sweden, a biologist has developed a method for freeze-drying dead bodies. Besides purportedly being environmentally friendly, freeze-drying is also said to be inexpensive, it makes corpses light and easy to transport, and it renders them harmless to work with.[57] The parallels between the new methods of handling dead bodies are striking. Advocates of cremation allied their cause with the vast discourse on hygiene that prevailed in all areas of society during Sweden's intense period of modernization around 1900. Today, proponents of the freeze-drying method have instead linked themselves with (or sprung out of) the contemporary discourse on environmental issues.

Unanswered Questions

The cremationists' conceptual agenda contains other interesting lines of thought that merit further study. One of these is the idea that the human body is part of the natural cycle of life and that after death it is returned to the environment through cremation. The idea seems odd—why take such a circuitous route, using an energy-intensive, technical, and artificial process to return the body to the environment?

It would also be interesting to study general attitudes toward cremation. For those who were relatively radical or who wanted to be modern, the symbolic value of cremation was certainly positive. Yet many others perceived cremation as negative and threatening. Those who lived in an area with a crematorium were more positive toward cremation, but there is more to it than that. The subject of cremation was ideologically charged. Choosing cremation signaled that a person held certain opinions and had made lifestyle choices.

The perception of cremation changed over time. One of the Nordic Museum's informants, who grew up next to a cemetery in the city of Gothenburg, captured this development. She described her parents as "very religious," and when her father died in 1929, cremation was not considered: "Cremation was very rare at that time. There was a crematorium at the East Cemetery, but in the circles to which my parents belonged, it was viewed as almost heathen." Her mother lived until 1965, and her final plea was: "You aren't going to burn me, are you?" The informant regarded her parents' view as old-fashioned, and she concluded: "Today cremation is very common, and no one in our day, or at least very few, see it as heathen, especially since we live in a big city, with its limited space."[58] In a typical manner, the values-based resistance to cremation by the older, church-going generation was replaced by the more pragmatic attitudes of a younger generation. The idea that cremation was a heathen or anti-Christian custom has lived on in some quarters, however. As late as 1989, a priest in the Church of Sweden from the province of Småland published an anti-cremation pamphlet.[59]

The writings of cremationists give the impression that opponents of cremation were primarily judgmental traditionalists from within the church, but it was not that simple. Even those who did not actively oppose the new practice might have doubts and reservations in the face of the unknown. For someone unfamiliar with the custom of cremation, having a deceased loved one cremated was not a viable alternative; that which is foreign could be perceived as frightening. Early on, a plethora of myths grew up about what went on in crematoriums.

One of the best-known myths, which the cremationists tried to rebuff repeatedly, with exasperation, was that the body sits itself upright in the incinerator.[60] In a book on modern legends, folklorist Bengt af Klintberg recounts another cremation myth, about a family who regularly received packages of food from relatives in the United States. The packages often contained such modern novelties as cake mixes. Once, they received a package containing only a carton of grayish-white powder, without instructions. The family tried to use the contents to bake a cake, but it did not turn out well and tasted bad. Some time later a letter arrived, explaining that the package had contained the ashes of an aunt.[61] Modern legends about cremation and crematoriums vary from country to country and follow local patterns of cremation. In the United Kingdom, where the casket glides out of the crematorium chapel on a conveyor belt at the end of the ceremony, funeral guests often imagine that they see flames and hear the roar of the fire as it passes through the doorway.[62]

Cremation did not, as the cremationists imagined, put an end to fearful fantasies about what might happen to the bodies of the deceased. The risk of being buried alive did disappear, and with it the legends about people who sat up in their coffins during their wake, gave birth to children while lying in a mortuary, or desperately tried to claw their way out of a buried coffin. Venetia Newall, who has written about the folklore of cremation in the United Kingdom, also points out that there are no ghost stories about persons who have been cremated. The idea of a ghost seems to require that the deceased person's body is not destroyed so quickly.[63] Nonetheless, the myths and legends surrounding earth burial were replaced by new ones about the practice of cremation.

Another unanswered question that deserves attention concerns the relationship of cremationists to racial thinking and Germanicism in general and to Nazi Germany in particular. The Swedish cremation movement included persons with highly varied political preferences, and nothing indicates that the members of the movement sympathized with Nazism to any degree. However, some of the movement's prominent figures, especially Gustav Schlyter and Oscar Övden, had positive attitudes toward Germany and were sometimes anti-Semitic. Schlyter's mystical view of the world included ideas of the superiority of the Germanic race, of flaming swastikas, and the belief that cremation in some obscure way could aid in the campaign against racial degeneration.[64] Övden, for his part, had contact with the Grossdeutscher Feuerbestattungsverein in Berlin. Heinz Zeiss, the chair of this huge German cremation association, thanked Övden for sending him copies of the journal *Ignis:*

> Following the campaign in Poland, I read with curiosity the isssues of *Ignis* for September–December 1939. Again and again, I had to put my hand to my helmet; despite my poor knowledge of your mother tongue, reading *Ignis* has for me been a true pleasure.

Övden proudly recounted this missive in the 1941 edition of *Meddelanden.*[65] He maintained his contact with the German cremationists throughout World War II.

From Radical to Conventional

The introduction and gradual acceptance of cremation in Sweden occurred in conjunction with the development of modern Swedish society. The membership of the Swedish Cremation Society changed character over time. From the beginning, cremation was a cause championed by members of the elite bourgeoisie, or rather the more radical representatives of this group. The society attracted famous, respected, and sometimes controversial members of the Swedish population: doctors, engineers, publishers, and politicians, as well as industrialists and businessmen. Among the most famous members were feminist writer Ellen Key, publicist and anatomist Gustaf Retzius, industrialist L. O. Smith, and Social Democratic leader Hjalmar Branting. The *Meddelanden* published membership lists, names of board members of the growing number of local branches, cremation statistics, and lists of famous persons who had been cremated. These lists served as an argument in and of themselves, a rhetoric of lists that conveys the belief that factual details could speak volumes on their own.[66]

In the 1920s, the local branch of the Cremation Society in the city of Gothenburg counted the influential editor Torgny Segerstedt among its members, and the membership roster in Stockholm included the well-known architect Ragnar Östberg. Thus the society was not a peripheral phenomenon that attracted only eccentrics. Rather, its members were often persons who played important roles in the social and cultural changes sweeping across Sweden in the decades just prior to and after the turn of the twentieth century. The Swedish Cremation Society was one of many groups of that era whose members were actively involved in a broad range of other contemporary issues. It shared members with the Swedish Touring Club, the Fredrika Bremer Association, the Swedish Society for the Protection of Animals, the Technology Society, and many more. Many of the society's members were also professionally engaged in the processes that were changing the foundations of Swedish society.

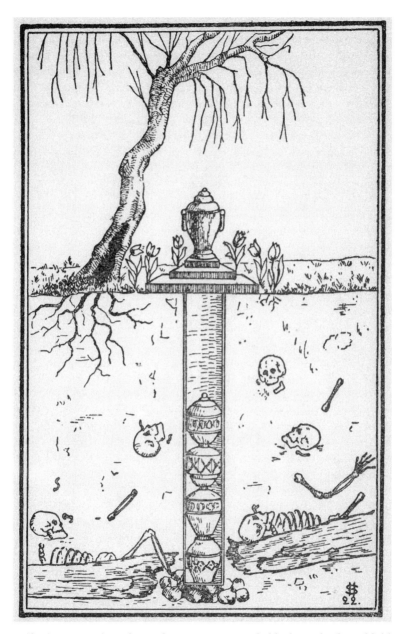

Figure 49. A cross-section of a modern urn grave, probably drawn by Gustaf Schlyter's son, Hans (ca. 1920). The neatly organized cremation urns are contrasted against the chaos that prevails in the surrounding soil of the cemetery. From Gustaf Schlyter, *Die Feuerbestattung und ihre kulturelle Bedeutung: Der Tempel des Friedens* (Leipzig, 1922), 332 (see also 342). Duplication: Kungl. biblioteket - National Library of Sweden.

Initially, the cremationist cause was championed mostly by the wealthy. It was also a men's cause. Very few women joined the society during its first decades, and even fewer women were active members. The active female members were often married to men who were driving forces in the society, such as Ragnhild Schlyter and Elma Övden. As might be expected and thought suitable in that era, these two women worked with cremation's "softer" aesthetic aspects, such as decorations and the layout of outdoor columbaria. The "hard" political, economic, and technical issues were addressed by male members. However, there were exceptions. For example, during the 1920s the local Stockholm branch counted one of Sweden's first female doctors, the controversial Ada Nilsson, among its members.[67] From the 1920s on, an increasing number of women became members of the society.

Even persons of middle- and working-class backgrounds joined in increasing numbers. The 1930s in particular saw a large influx of laborers after the society established its own insurance plan in 1931. In fact, the society was not a "movement" in the true sense of the word until the great swelling of the ranks that occurred in the 1930s.[68] The type of person who joined varied depending on geographic area as well. Local branches in some of Sweden's highly industrialized communities experienced rapid growth. For example, in the town of Sandviken, the number of cremations performed skyrocketed after the town built a crematorium in 1935.[69]

In the 1880s, the choice of cremation was considered extreme. It was a choice associated with radicalism, liberalism, and a critical view of established religious orthodoxy and traditional, homogeneous society. It was an individual choice that indicated a seemingly rational relationship with death. Yet a pro-cremation stance also signaled a new, specifically modern sensitivity to the disintegration of the dead body. Cremationist publications did not present the romantic, poetic relationship with decay of Baudelaire or the Swedish poet Stagnelius. Further, the image of the decaying body was not used to inspire philosophical thoughts about one's own mortality, as had been the case during the sixteenth century. Instead, the dead body had become a threat to emotions, health, society, and culture. This threat had to be disarmed, something best achieved with the help of purifying flames.[70] The cremationists' feeling of distaste toward decay is captured in a 1922 drawing of an urn grave shown in cross-section (see figure 49).

With the assistance of engineers, the cremationists created a technology for dealing with the problems associated with death. The potentially dangerous body was deposited in an incinerator, and out came a harmless substance. The ash was sterile and could not hurt anyone; it could not infect people or come back to haunt the living. This new funeral technique, regarded as extreme in its early years, came to be viewed as normal. Modern society and the modern funeral technique had found one another.

In 1929, when Oscar Övden called cremation "the funeral practice of the future," he did not know how close he was to the truth. That same year, the city of Helsingborg dedicated its crematorium, the fifth built in Sweden since the first small, rather provisory facility was built in Stockholm in 1887. A wave of crematorium building took place in Sweden in the 1930s, but only 4.5 percent of the dead were cremated. After more than five decades, the cremation movement had not convinced the Swedish people of the advantages of cremation. Subsequently, however, the numbers rose quickly. In 2002, 70 percent of dead Swedes and over 90 percent of dead Stockholmers were cremated.[71]

The cremationist propaganda of those first decades tended to be provocatively radical and anti-church and, at the same time, romantically religious. However, cremation did not fully gain acceptance in Sweden until those characteristics were eliminated. In addition, it helped that new crematoria were designed as regular funeral chapels and that the practice of cremation was packaged in a clear ritual form.

The introduction of cremation modernized the handling of dead bodies. The interwar period in Sweden was a time of democratic breakthroughs. Values promoted by members of Sweden's radical bourgeoisie in the late nineteenth century began to find more widespread acceptance. In an increasingly prosperous Sweden, the cremation movement's key concepts of hygiene, aesthetics, and technology could be embraced by a growing number of people from different levels of society. At the same time that social conditions were ripe for a new funeral practice, cremation had matured to a point where society could now accept it.

I regard the crematorium as a symbol of modern society's perception of death. The crematorium houses two aspects of death: the practical side, represented by components such as cold storage rooms and elevators, and the emotional or spiritual side, represented by the chapel, a room for ritual. These two aspects meet in the crematorium building. Within its walls, the unsightly and unhygienic corpse is transformed into an emotionally and hygienically acceptable substance. In the crematorium building, the body is purified by flames.

The dead body is perceived as intimidating and unclean in modernity. Why? What is it that makes a corpse so threatening? Chapter 7 includes a discussion of the practical and ritual ways in which modern people tried to take control of the dead body's menacing aspects.

Chapter Seven

Abjection and Modern Rituals

The dead human body's unclear status between being and not being makes the living uneasy. To avoid such feelings, we seek solutions to the threatening liminality of the corpse. Destroying the corpse through cremation is one attempt at a solution; binding its feet so it cannot walk the earth again is another. Each era and each culture has its own ways of dealing with this problem.[1]

One explanation for the ever-present fear of (and fascination with) dead bodies is that they are neither objects nor subjects. To use Julia Kristeva's terminology, they are "abjects." The abject has dual status: it is both and neither; either and or; it disgusts and attracts; it is obscure and destroys established order; it is a passage and a place for threshold experiences. The sense of disgust over the unclean or over food, filth, garbage, and especially corpses is a reaction related to the demarcation of boundaries, which Kristeva refers to as "abjection."

> If dung signifies the other side of the border, the place where I am not and which permits me to be, the corpse, the most sickening of wastes, is a border that has encroached upon everything. . . . In that compelling, raw, insolent thing in the morgue's full sunlight, in that thing that no longer matches and therefore no longer signifies anything, I behold the breaking down of a world that has erased its borders: fainting away. The corpse, seen without God and outside of science, is the utmost of abjection. It is death infecting life. Abject. . . . Imaginary uncanniness and real threat, it beckons to us and ends up engulfing us.[2]

The corpse—the abject—challenges the identity of anyone confronting it. At the same time, it sets down the boundaries of the self and culture. In the face of the terrifying phenomenon of death, the living body becomes clearly defined as living.[3] In passing, Kristeva also points out the two systems of thought that have been used to explain and deal with the threat the dead body poses: religion and science.

Yet the abject nature of the corpse does not explain why the ways of dealing with its ambiguous nature have changed throughout history. The answer to that question, I argue, must be that the variable roles and meanings of death and dead bodies are responses to shifting, culturally constituted needs. If death disturbs and threatens an established social order and if ritual acts serve, among other things, the function of creating a new order, then studies of death practices will inform us about the culture and the society being studied.[4] People with different worldviews and forms of social organization generate different death and burial customs. Surrounding the dead with ritual acts is a general need, while the specific forms of these acts change; people in modernity created the rituals they wanted while transforming existing traditions. This study is thus a contribution not only to the history of death customs but also to the history of modernity. With Sweden's modernization around the turn of the twentieth century, attitudes toward death, like many other things, changed profoundly. The previous chapters have described such attitudes by empirically examining some of the changing ways people have handled dead bodies. In conclusion, this chapter discusses change, continuity, and the consequences of modernity as they pertain to the handling of dead human bodies.

This study is not the first to demonstrate differences between "traditional" and modern ways of relating to death. As chapter 1 explained, many existing studies have pointed out these differences by contrasting older customs and traditions with newer ones. This volume has used case studies to explore the concrete ways some such changes took place. Since the focus of this book is on the dead body, I have omitted many aspects such as dying, grief, and conceptions of what happens on "the other side."

It is often said that in modern society death has been rationalized, medicalized, secularized, individualized, and commercialized. This view is implicitly critical of the relationship between modern culture and death, contrasting it with the supposedly "natural" attitudes of pre-modern society. What is revealed is a nostalgic fantasy of an imagined social unity that is supposed to have been destroyed by modern society. But these "-izations" are also prominent characteristics of modernization, and it would be remarkable if they had *not* influenced the status of death in modern culture. Thus the modernity-critical view of the cultural history of death contains an implicit idealization of the customs and traditions of the old society. In my opinion, this critical stance toward modernity should be regarded with skepticism.[5]

The old customs in nineteenth-century Swedish agrarian society demonstrate that death was a problem people tried to deal with through ritual acts. For example, as shown by Louise Hagberg and others, people feared the supernatural trouble a corpse could cause. Corpses also smelled bad and were damaged by rats—repulsive facts people sought to prevent by various methods. Funerals were important social events, but they were also manifestations of social status and positions of power. The funerals of the poor and destitute and those who had committed suicide were demonstrations of those persons' social disenfranchisement.

Against this background, a feature of modernization such as the establishment of better storage places for dead bodies awaiting burial cannot be regarded as a concealment of death. Rather, it was a way of using modern building and transportation methods to solve a real problem that had more dimensions than purely hygienic ones. Further, using the services of a professional funeral director did not necessarily indicate a desire to push the problem of death out of one's personal life. Instead, it could be a way of doing something special for the deceased—treating the person in accordance with the new modern era. The leveling of obvious social differences in cemeteries and funeral services was also an active attempt to change conditions for the better, for both the deceased and the living.

After analyzing the meanings of the new ways of dealing with death in modernity, I have found no reason to join the chorus of those critical of modernity. Among the phenomena I have studied, some were fading within Swedish culture, while others were on the rise. Pathology, in all its forms, had come to stay, as had autopsies and other methods of examining organs and tissues from corpses. Anatomy as a field of research and education experienced a great upswing around the turn of the twentieth century but later diminished in importance. Cremation as an alternative funeral practice was definitely gaining acceptance, as were mortuaries and professional funeral directors. On their way to disappearing were the practices of local women washing and clothing corpses and the customs of viewing the dead body and keeping the deceased in the home prior to burial.

The custom of photographing the dead and keeping the photographs as mementos reached a high point in the decades just prior to and after 1900. The same is true of displays of dead bodies and body parts in medical anatomy museums and commercial wax museums. On the threshold of the modern era, it was thus common to exhibit death and examine it in many forms: as a visual object within the cultures of science and spectacle, as part of the funeral ritual of viewing the deceased, and in memorial photographs and pictorial representations of dead persons in the illustrated press.

In modern Sweden, most of these forms of meeting with death, or with the corpse as its representative, have disappeared. They were specific to and characteristic of the culture of the late nineteenth and early twentieth centuries. In the late-modern twenty-first century, death is still visible in the mass media and popular culture, although not in the same way as in previous eras. Today, impersonal dead bodies are shown, such as victims of war and violence, most often from distant places. For example, when the famous Swedish children's author Astrid Lindgren died in late winter 2002, no newspapers ran deathbed portraits of her. Doing so would have been unimaginable and perceived as offensive. At around the same time, however, Sweden's largest daily newspaper ran a press photograph showing two soldiers posing with a trophy at their feet: a human being whom they had just fatally shot in one of the bloodiest and most violent conflicts in history.[6]

In nineteenth-century Swedish agrarian society, the unclean and liminal nature of the corpse was dealt with in ways fundamentally different from those employed in modern society. The dead body was ritually washed and dressed; it was made attractive and shown in a decorated room. People followed the corpse to the grave in a procession. The deceased could be hindered from walking the earth again by sticking needles into his or her heels. These acts involved many people, and everything had to be done in certain predetermined ways to guarantee both the welfare of the deceased in the next world and the safety of the living in this one.

In the transition to modern society, by contrast, the danger and uncleanliness of the corpse were presented as a hygienic problem. This problem was dealt with in supposedly rational ways, supported by science and technology. The unclean corpse was kept separate from the living and was disposed of in ways similar to other filth. It became unhygienic to keep the corpse at home prior to burial, which necessitated the construction of corpse storage rooms and mortuaries. The disorderliness and stench of cemeteries were eliminated, and cemeteries were arranged as pleasant parks. With the new cremation technology, industrial methods were used to transform the dead body from a potential source of contagion to a harmless, packaged product. The problems of death and decay were now discussed in scientific and medical terms rather than religious ones.

Dead bodies could be used as sources of scientific knowledge and thus be of benefit to the living. This was certainly not new, but it was a controversial attitude toward the dead body that found greater acceptance in modernity and can be related to the general breakthrough of scientific attitudes in modern society. Previously, the corpse was sometimes perceived as dangerous in a supernatural way. In the modern era, the corpse was also considered a potential risk for the living, but not because it might walk the earth again and pull the living down into the grave. Instead, the danger a corpse posed was defined scientifically: it could cause harm through bacteria and poisons that develop during the process of decay.

In my opinion, these modern perceptions about the uncleanliness of the dead body still have symbolic aspects, and this perceived uncleanliness is dealt with in ritual ways that are suited to modern society. Transporting the dead body to a hygienic mortuary can be viewed as one such example. As Jonas Frykman put it, it is "too simple to believe that ideas of cleanliness were nothing but a result of increased knowledge about the origins of disease. It is also too simple to believe that the war against bacteria was waged solely for medical motives."[7]

It is difficult to distinguish between practical and ritual aspects of death. I have tried to avoid falling into the trap of overemphasizing the ritual functions of acts in the past and the practical functions of (or rational explanations for) modern behaviors. Modern death customs have not diminished the corpse's liminal and threatening nature. The problem remains and cannot be controlled rationally because a corpse is not simply refuse but the abject remains of a human being. Instead of claiming that death has been pushed aside or hidden in modernity, I would say that death has been cleaned away from everyday life. In an era when Sweden was cleansed of many other sorts of perceived filth, even death was sanitized. The physical presence of death in the form of dead human bodies was perceived as detrimental, unmodern. With the help of hospitals, mortuaries, corpse sheds, funeral homes, and crematoriums, corpses were removed from everyday life. For moderns, this cleanliness liberated Swedes from the backwardness and filthy conditions of earlier eras. One of the most important elements in the modernization of death was its incorporation into this culture of cleanliness.[8]

Dead bodies were also removed from doctors' cabinets. Dusty anatomical museum displays were packed up and stashed away, discarded, or burned. In Sweden, this cleanup campaign seems to have been extremely thorough. Old collections of anatomical and pathological preparations are preserved with pride in many other countries. These collections are regarded as valuable, both didactically for today's medical students and as objects of medical history. In countries neighboring Sweden, such as Finland and Estonia, people still take photographs of deceased family members. Why not in Sweden? Have Swedes developed a particularly strong sensitivity to the physical presence of death? Is the modern ideology of hygiene more powerful in Sweden and applied more strongly to death than it is in neighboring countries?

Abjection, the sense of disgust toward dead bodies, played a prominent role in the cremationists' arguments. They found the imagined horrors of decay in the grave unbearable. Cremation offered a solution to this problem. Now, the scientific view of the human body has become normal, and an autopsy is usually accepted and sometimes even desired by survivors. Although researchers, forensic pathologists, and laboratory assistants who work with dead bodies are sometimes considered disgusting or bizarre their work is a regular part of modern death practice, one step in the series of events that follow a death.[9] To surviving family members, the body of a deceased loved one is always more than a piece of dead biological material. Why, then, do we willingly allow the deceased to be cut up and analyzed down to the smallest cell? The person who agrees to an autopsy makes the supposition that something more is to be known than the simple fact that the loved one is dead and believes that this knowledge is important. Discovering the cause of death, or the physical events that led up to it, has emerged as part of the process of (re)establishing meaning and social order after someone dies. The cruelty of death might be diminished by the medical explanation. If so, the pathological laboratory is a ritual room for the creation of order, explanation, and reconstruction. The scientific method is one of history's many culture-specific attempts to deal with the problem of the dead body and the threat it poses to life, in a way suited to modern society.

Compared to the rites of passage that structured death and burial in previous times, the rites of *transition* and *incorporation* diminished during the period I have studied, while the *separation* grew more prominent. The separation of the deceased from the world of the living became more definite through autopsies, storage in mortuaries, professional funeral care, and cremation. During the twentieth century, this tendency was further emphasized when the dying (but still living) were moved into hospitals and other care facilities. The ritual of the funeral procession thus lost its cultural significance in modernity. In earlier eras, funerals were charged with the belief that the deceased live on in a new fellowship on the other side of death, whether in heaven, hell, or the world below the graveyard. Increasingly, funeral rites were instead regarded as supporting the survivors in managing their grief, and the need for rituals was explained in psychological rather than religious terms.

This book has depicted the changing ways of handling dead bodies in Sweden around the turn of the twentieth century as manifestations of the transition to modernity. It has shown that beliefs and death practices were complex and variable during this specific historical period. Each society or culture develops ways of dealing with death suited to prevailing worldviews and ways of living. When they no longer fill a need, ritual acts lose their meaning and die out. New rites come into being in conjunction with changing social conditions and cultural concepts. Not even the moderns could do without rituals, so they invented their own.

Notes

Chapter One

Epigraph. Peter Metcalf and Richard Huntington, *Celebrations of Death: The Anthropology of Mortuary Ritual* (Cambridge: Cambridge University Press, 1991 [1979]), 24.

1.   Among the best-known and most influential works on the history of death are those by French historian Philippe Ariès. See note 2. Swiss-American psychiatrist Elisabeth Kübler-Ross's writings on death and dying attracted much attention and were conducive to the formation of the research field known as thanatology. See, for example, *On Death and Dying* (New York: Macmillan, 1969). Geoffrey Gorer's article "The Pornography of Death" (*Encounter,* October 1955) defined death as the taboo of modern times and has been quoted ever since. More important for my work were: (1) French historian of mentalities Michel Vovelle's *La mort et l'Occident de 1300 à nos jours* (Paris: Gallimard, 1983), which is less sweeping and more focused on historically specific *changes* in the history of death than Ariès's work; (2) Polish-British sociologist Zygmunt Bauman's *Mortality, Immortality, and Other Life Strategies* (Cambridge, UK: Polity, 1992), which philosophically discusses (modern) culture as a defense against the fearful knowledge of our mortality; (3) British sociologist Tony Walter's *The Revival of Death* (London: Routledge, 1994), which deals with the late-modern discourse on death; and (4) Metcalf and Huntington's *Celebrations of Death,* which is a rich anthropological work that analyzes a wide variety of cultural manifestations linked with death worldwide.

2.   Philippe Ariès, *The Hour of Our Death* (Oxford: Oxford University Press, 1991) [*Homme devant la mort* (Paris: Éditions du Seuil, 1977)], 612–14 (quote on 613–14). See also Ariès's *Western Attitudes toward Death: From the Middle Ages to the Present* (Baltimore: Johns Hopkins University Press, 1974) [*Essais sur l'histoire de la mort en Occident* (Paris: Éditions du Seuil, 1971)]; *Images of Man and Death* (Cambridge, MA: Harvard University Press, 1985) [*Images de l'homme devant la mort* (Paris: Éditions du Seuil, 1983)].

3.   Ariès, *Hour of Our Death,* 614. Although Ariès claims that this utopian future without a fear of death is the goal of "a small elite of anthropologists, psychologists, and sociologists," it is obviously also his own dream.

4.   Vovelle, *La mort et l'Occident de 1300,* introduction, especially 11–12.

5.   Swedish ethnologist Lynn Åkesson even suggests the possibility that we fear death less now than people did in other times. Åkesson, *Mellan levande och döda: Föreställningar om kropp och ritual* (Stockholm: Natur och kultur, 1997), 12. Also see Åkesson, "Döda kroppars budskap," in *Kroppens tid: Om samspelet mellan kropp, identitet och samhälle,* ed. Lynn Åkesson and Susanne Lundin (Stockholm: Natur och kultur, 1996); Åkesson and Lundin, "Att skapa liv och utforska död," *Kulturella perspektiv* 1 (1995).

6.   On the history of suicide in Sweden, see Anders Ekström, *Dödens exempel: Självmordstolkningar i svenskt 1800-tal genom berättelsen om Otto Landgren* (Stockholm: Atlantis, 2000); Arne Jarrick, *Hamlets fråga: En svensk självmordshistoria* (Stockholm: Norstedts, 2000); Birgitta Odén, Bodil E.B. Persson, and Yvonne Maria Werner, *Den frivilliga döden: Samhällets hantering av självmord i historiskt perspektiv* (Stockholm: Cura and FRN, 1998); Ann-Sofie Ohlander, " 'den smärtsamma oro, vilken bragt honom ända till ledsnad vid livet': Synen på självmordet i Sverige från medeltid till 1900-tal," in *Kärlek, död och frihet: Historiska uppsatser om människovärde och livsvillkor i Sverige* (Stockholm: Norstedts, 1986). On dead children in art, see Karin Sidén, *Den ideala barndomen: Studier i det stormaktstida barnporträttets ikonografi och funktion* (Stockholm: Raster, 2001), chapter 5. See also Metcalf and Huntington, *Celebrations of Death,* part 3: "The Royal Corpse and the Body Politic"; Mårten Snickare, *Enväldets riter: Kungliga fester och ceremonier i gestaltning av Nicodemus Tessin den yngre* (Stockholm: Raster, 1999).

7.   Metcalf and Huntington, *Celebrations of Death.* The book's perspective is global and comparative and takes its point of departure in the extremely diversified ways of handling dead bodies around the world. Huntington and Metcalf utilize and discuss earlier critical anthropological research on the subject while also using their own field studies.

8.   Arnold van Gennep, *Les rites de passage: Etude systématique des rites* (Paris: É. Nourry, 1909).

9.   Even family members of the deceased undergo rites of passage—they take on special roles during the grieving period and are later inducted into their social context in their new roles.

10.   Van Gennep used the term "liminality" to indicate the state in which a person finds him- or herself during the transition phase. Victor Turner broadened this concept to include states outside or on the periphery of everyday life, and he pointed out that liminality often is (or may easily become) a holy state. Turner further maintained that entire societies may be characterized as liminal during a transition between different social structures. See Turner, *Dramas, Fields, and Metaphors: Symbolic Action in Human Society* (Ithaca, NY: Cornell University Press, 1974), 47, 231–32.

11.   Regarding rituals, order, and meaning, see Victor Turner, *The Anthropology of Performance* (New York: PAJ, 1986).

12.   I have consciously expressed myself in a general way. For studies of ideas connected with the magical powers of dead bodies, see Metcalf and Huntington, *Celebrations of Death;* Louise Hagberg, *När döden gästar: Svenska folkseder och svensk folktro i samband med död och begravning* (Stockholm: Wahlström och Widstrand, 1937); Yvonne Verdier, *Façons de dire, façons de faire: La laveuse, la couturière, la cuisinière* (Paris: Gallimard, 1979) [I have used the Swedish translation *Tvätterskan, kokerskan, sömmerskan: Livet i en fransk by genom tre kvinnoyrken* (Stockholm: Atlantis, 1981)]; Ulrika Wolf-Knuts, "Liktvättning—ett kvinnoarbete," in *Budkavlen* (Åbo: Åbo Akademi, 1983). This theme is discussed in chapter 4.

13.   Mary Douglas, *Purity and Danger: An Analysis of the Concepts of Pollution and Taboo* (London: Routledge, 1996 [1966]).

14.   Ibid., 2–6. Douglas's study covers "primitive cultures" (those without written language), but this reasoning may be applied to other contexts. Douglas also separates the hygienic aspects, which change with one's level of knowledge, from the

symbolic and conventional views of filth (7). I am convinced, however, that even the hygienic views contain symbolism and not just rational thinking.

15. See ibid., 122–24.

16. For support of an eclectic approach to research, see Ludmilla Jordanova, *Sexual Visions: Images of Gender in Science and Medicine between the Eighteenth and Twentieth Centuries* (Madison: University of Wisconsin Press, 1989), 6.

17. In recent decades, anthropological research has inspired many historians, including me. It is not always the latest developments in anthropological research that are of relevance for historians; rather, it is primarily the open-minded and self-reflexive way anthropologists relate to and analyze culture.

18. Culture is studied in many academic disciplines (cultural studies, ethnology, anthropology, sociology, archaeology, philosophy, media and communications studies, as well as in the various historical disciplines). "Culture" is a concept that is under discussion, which has by turns been given very broad and more limited definitions (for a good overview, see Robert Bocock, "The Cultural Formations of Modern Society," in *Modernity: An Introduction to Modern Societies*, ed. S. Hall, D. Held, D. Hubert, and K. Thompson [Cambridge, MA: Blackwell, 1996]). I use Geertz's concept because it is concrete and usable. Clifford Geertz, "Thick Description: Toward an Interpretive Theory of Cultures," in *The Interpretation of Cultures* (London: Fontana, 1993 [1973]).

19. Geertz, "Thick Description," 14 et passim.

20. Ibid., 17.

21. Here Geertz is clearly polemic toward anthropologists who have a too-broad concept of culture and toward structuralists generally.

22. Geertz, "Thick Description," 30. Geertz has been criticized, discussed, and utilized in other ways than the one I employ here—I have chosen to emphasize aspects that have been useful for my study.

23. This discussion of Ricoeur's view on history is based mostly on the essay "Le temps raconté," *Revue de Métaphysique et de Morale* 4 (1984). I used the Swedish translation "Den berättade tiden" in *Från text till handling: En antologi om hermeneutik* (Lund: Symposion, 1988 [1986]).

24. Ricoeur, "Le temps raconté," 209. The main difference between the work of the historian and that of the novelist is that the historian, bound to the reality of the past, only creates reconstructions and is not, like the writer, free to create his or her own fantasy world that can have any sort of relationship with the real world. In contrast to the novel, the historian's constructions seek to be re-constructions of the past, according to Ricoeur. He called the historian "our representative for memory" in that he or she "stands in debt to the past, owes a debt of gratitude to the dead" (221–23).

25. Ibid., 219–22.

26. Ibid., 224. According to Ricoeur, the work of the historian is characterized by our understanding of the past as simultaneously absent from and (through historical traces) present in our time. Historical research, however, contains a problematic "relation of representation," and there are many different ideas about how historical narration should relate to historical reality. Ricoeur suggests that we should "attempt to approach the problem tropologically," and he refers to Hayden White and his books *Metahistory: The Historical Imagination in Nineteenth Century Europe* (Baltimore:

Johns Hopkins University Press, 1978) and *Tropics of Discourse: Essays in Cultural Criticism* (Baltimore: Johns Hopkins University Press, 1978).

27. Geertz, "Thick Description," 11.

28. Ricoeur, "Le temps raconté," 224–26. In characterizing the historian's knowledge, Ricoeur refers to Leopold Ranke's old and often-criticized goal for historical writing: to depict something "wie es eigentlich gewesen." The emphasis here, according to Ricoeur, is not on the word *eigentlich* but rather on the word *wie*, which means an important shift of meaning: seeing histories not as objective representations of past reality but as narratives based on subjective interpretation.

29. Philip Brey discusses the history and contents of theories of modernity in a particularly clarifying and useful way in "Theorizing Modernity and Technology," in *Modernity and Technology*, ed. T. J. Misa, P. Brey, and A. Feenberg (Cambridge, MA: MIT Press, 2003), 33–62. For some central texts on modernity, see Marshall Berman, *All That Is Solid Melts into Air: The Experience of Modernity* (New York: Simon and Schuster, 1982); Anthony Giddens, *The Consequences of Modernity* (Stanford: Stanford University Press, 1990); Jürgen Habermas, *The Structural Transformation of the Public Sphere* (Cambridge, MA: MIT Press, 1989); Fredric Jameson, *A Singular Modernity: Essay on the Ontology of the Present* (London: Verso, 2002); Bruno Latour, *We Have Never Been Modern* (Cambridge, MA: Harvard University Press, 1993 [1991]); *Modernity: An Introduction to Modern Societies*, ed. S. Hall, D. Held, D. Hubert, and K. Thompson (Cambridge, MA: Blackwell, 1996); Bryan S. Turner, *Theories of Modernity and Postmodernity* (London: Sage, 1990); Max Weber, *The Protestant Ethic and the Spirit of Capitalism* (New York: Scribner's, 1958 [1905]). For a study of social movements, sociology, and modernity in Sweden, see Håkan Thörn, *Modernitet, sociologi och sociala rörelser* (Göteborg: Sociologiska institutionen, Göteborgs universitet, 1997).

30. In *The Culture of Time and Space, 1880–1918* (Cambridge: Harvard University Press, 2003 [1983]), Stephen Kern brings to life the way the realization of such technological innovations influenced people's experience of time and space (the book is an excellent study of modernity and modernization in which the author barely mentions these concepts). For a study of how new techniques of illumination influenced people's life-worlds, see Jan Garnert, *Anden i lampan: Etnologiska perspektiv på ljus och mörker* (Stockholm: Carlssons, 1993). See also *Modernity and Technology*, ed. Misa, Brey, and Feenberg.

31. The term "life-world" is used in sociology influenced by phenomenological philosophy. For a discussion of the differences between discursive and life-world practices, see Thörn, *Modernitet*, 146–48.

32. Roger Qvarsell, "Inledning," in *I framtidens tjänst: Ur folkhemmets idéhistoria*, ed. Roger Qvarsell (Stockholm: Gidlunds, 1986), 18–20.

33. Gunnar Broberg and Mattias Tydén, *Oönskade i folkhemmet: Rashygien och sterilisering i Sverige* (Stockholm: Gidlunds, 1991); Karin Johannisson, *Den mörka kontinenten: Kvinnan, medicinen och fin-de-siècle* (Stockholm: Norstedts, 1994); Johannisson, *Kroppens tunna skal: Sex essäer om kropp, historia och kultur* (Stockholm: Norstedts, 1997); among works by Roger Qvarsell, see *Vårdens idéhistoria* (Stockholm: Carlssons, 1991) and *Utan vett och vilja: Om synen på brottslighet och sinnessjukdom* (Stockholm: Carlssons, 1993). See also Bengt Erik Eriksson and Eva Palmblad, *Kropp och politik: Hälsoupplysning som samhällsspegel från 30-tal till 90-tal* (Stockholm: Carlssons, 1995).

34. Kjell Jonsson, "En nybadad renrasig svensk på ett blankpolerat furugolv i ett hus utan löss i ett genomskinligt samhälle där vetenskapen ser till att fabrikerna tillverkar foträta skor och ingen är så dum att han på fotboll glor—Hjalmar Öhrvalls person-, bostads-, mental-, och rashygien såsom samhällsvision," in *I framtidens tjänst*, 104–6.

35. Sverker Sörlin, "Utopin i verkligheten: Ludvig Nordström och det moderna Sverige," in *I framtidens tjänst*, 187.

36. Kjell Jonsson has written about the demarcation between the respective spheres of science and religion in *Vid vetandets gräns: Om skiljelinjen mellan naturvetenskap och metafysik i svensk kulturdebatt 1870–1920* (Lund: Arkiv, 1987) and in *Harmoni eller konflikt? En idéhistorisk introduktion till förhållandet mellan vetenskap och religion i Västerlandet* (Stockholm: Carlssons, 1991). For more on the role of science in Swedish modernity, see Nils Runeby, *Teknikerna, vetenskapen och kulturen: Ingenjörsundervisning och ingenjörsorganisationer i 1870-talets Sverige* (Uppsala: Institutionen för idé- och lärdomshistoria, Uppsala universitet, 1976); Gunnar Eriksson, *Kartläggarna: Naturvetenskapens tillväxt och tillämpningar i det industriella genombrottets Sverige 1870–1914* (Umeå, Sweden: Umeå universitet, 1978); and the anthology *Vetenskapsbärarna: Naturvetenskapen i det svenska samhället 1880–1950*, ed. Sven Widmalm (Hedemora, Sweden: Gidlunds, 1999).

37. K. Robert V. Wikman, "Louise Hagberg †," in *Fataburen: Nordiska museets och Skansens årsbok* (Stockholm: 1945), 171.

38. Hagberg does not cite the source of her information, making it difficult to know if it can be trusted. After comparing Hagberg's reports with archival material at the Nordic Museum, I can state that she has reproduced this material correctly.

39. For a presentation of the history of Swedish ethnology, see Nils-Arvid Bringéus, *Människan som kulturvarelse: En introduktion till etnologin* (Stockholm: Carlssons, 1990 [1976]). For a thorough discussion of ethnological reports from Hagberg's time, see Agneta Lilja, *Föreställningen om den ideala uppteckningen: En studie av idé och praktik vid traditionssamlande arkiv—ett exempel från Uppsala 1914–1945* (Uppsala: Dialekt- och fornminnesarkivet, Uppsala universitet, 1996). See also two essays about Hagberg's work at the Nordic Museum: Hjördis Gustafsson, "Med karameller och entusiasm som trollmedel: Om folklivsforskaren Louise Hagbergs arbete på 1920-talet" (unpublished thesis, Stockholm, Institutet för folklivsforksning, Stockholms universitet, 1992); Susanne Nylund Skog, "Louise Hagberg som forskare och författare: En granskning av artikeln 'Julhalm och juldockor' och dess underlag" (unpublished thesis, Stockholm, Institutet för folklivsforksning, Stockholms universitet, 1993).

40. Hagberg, *När döden gästar*, 11.

41. On the Nordic Museum and its archives, see Karin Becker, "Picturing Our Past: An Archive Constructs a National Culture," *Journal of American Folklore* 105, no. 415 (1992); *Nordiska museet under 125 år*, ed. Hans Medelius, Bengt Nyström, and Elisabet Stavenow-Hidemark (Stockholm: Nordiska museets förlag, 1998).

42. Hagberg, *När döden gästar*, 12–13.

43. See in particular Nils-Arvid Bringéus, "Vår hållning till döden," in *Dödens riter*, ed. Kristina Söderpalm (Stockholm: Carlssons, 1994), in which new and old customs and ideas are juxtaposed. See also Bringéus, *Klockringningsseden i Sverige* (Stockholm: Nordiska Museets förlag, 1958.); "Vår hållning till döden, speglad genom begravninsseden förr och nu," in *Vår hållning till döden*, ed. Erik Bylund (Umeå, Sweden: CEWE-förlaget/Erik Bylund, 1983); and *Svensk begravningssed i historisk belysning*

(Fonus, 1983). Among other notable ethnological studies about death and burial is Mats Rehnberg, *Ljusen på gravarna och andra ljusseder: Nya traditioner under 1900-talet* (Stockholm: Nordiska museet, 1965); Hilding Pleijel, *Jordfästning i stillhet: Från samhällsstraff till privatceremoni: En samhällshistorisk studie* (Lund: Arken, 1983).

44. Bringéus, *Livets högtider* (Stockholm: LT, 1987).

45. Ibid., 254.

46. Bringéus deals with mainstream Swedish culture, dominated as it is by the Protestant traditions of the Church of Sweden. Catholics, Jews, Muslims, and other religious groups have their own customs, but they are not dealt with here.

47. Bringéus, *Livets högtider,* 176.

48. Bringéus, *Livets högtider,* 176–77. On women's mourning clothes at the Swedish royal court, see Angela Rundquist, "Hovfruntimret—ett nobelt yrkeskollektiv 1850–1900," *Livsrustkammaren* 17, no. 5–6 (1986).

49. For concentrated presentations of the history of anatomy and pathology, respectively, see Roger French, "The Anatomical Tradition," and Russell C. Maulitz, "The Pathological Tradition," both in *Companion Encyclopedia of the History of Medicine,* ed. W. F. Bynum and Roy Porter (London: Routledge, 1993). See also Russell C. Maulitz, *Morbid Appearances: The Anatomy of Pathology in the Early Nineteenth Century* (Cambridge: Cambridge University Press, 1987); Ruth Richardson, *Death, Dissection, and the Destitute* (London: Routledge and Kegan Paul, 1987); Michael Sappol, *A Traffic of Dead Bodies: Anatomy and Embodied Social Identity in Nineteenth-Century America* (Princeton: Princeton University Press, 2002).

50. Michel Foucault, *The Birth of the Clinic: An Archaeology of Medical Perception* (New York: Vintage Books, 1994 [1963]), 149. See also chapter 8, "Open up a Few Corpses," especially 143–45. On the history of the anatomo-clinical method in America, see John Harley Warner, *Against the Spirit of System: The French Impulse in Nineteenth-Century American Medicine* (Baltimore: Johns Hopkins University Press, 1998).

51. See Richardson, *Death, Dissection, and the Destitute;* Sappol, *A Traffic of Dead Bodies,* Helen MacDonald, *Human Remains: Episodes in Human Dissection* (Melbourne: Melbourne University Press, 2005).

52. Little has been written about the history of funeral directors. See, however, Anna Davidsson Bremborg, "Från stigmatisering till professionalisering? En studie av begravningsentreprenörer utifrån ett aktörsperspektiv" (unpublished master's thesis, Lund, Lund University, 2002) and her "Vem tar hand om den döda kroppen? Om genusarbetsfördelning på begravningsbyråer," in *Stigma, status och strategier: Genusperspektiv i religionsvetenskap,* ed. Catharina Raudvere (Lund: Studentlitteratur, 2002), and *Yrke: begravningsentreprenör: Om utanförskap, döda kroppar, riter och professionalisering* (Lund: Studentlitteratur, 2002). See also Hagberg, Verdier, and Wolf-Knuts.

53. In ethnological research, this genre of photography has mostly been used as a source of knowledge about casket styles and similar objects. However, the genre has been studied in its own right to some degree—see Sigurjón Baldur Hafsteinsson, "Post-mortem and Funeral Photography in Iceland," *History of Photography* (Spring 1999); Johanne Maria Jensen, *Gennem lys og skugger: Familiefotografier fra forrige århundrede til idag* (Herning, Denmark: Systime, 1994) and her "Livet og døden i familiealbumet," *Siden Saxo: Magasin for dansk historie* 4 (1995); Jay Ruby, *Secure the Shadow: Death and Photography in America* (Cambridge, MA: MIT Press 1995). My case study also required me to explore the history of photography, portrait history, and

research on the use of images in Swedish history. See Lena Johannesson, *Den mass-producerade bilden: Ur bildindustrialismens historia* (Stockholm: Carlssons, 1997 [1978]); Solfrid Söderlind, *Porträttbruk i Sverige 1840–1865* (Stockholm: Carlssons, 1994); Rolf Söderberg and Pär Rittsel, *Den svenska fotografins historia* (Stockholm: BonnierFakta, 1983).

Chapter Two

Epigraph. Salomon Eberhard Henschen, "Om den tekniska undersökningen af hjärnan: Några anmärkningar," in *Festskrift tillegnad direktören och öfverläkaren vid Sabbatsbergs sjukhus med doktorn F. W. Warfvinge vid fylda 60 år* (Stockholm, 1894), 185.

1. Gunnar Broberg, "En kulturanatom: Carl-Herman Hjortsjö," *Kulturanatomiska studier* (Lund: Lunds universitet, 2001), 68, photo on 69. This slogan is not unique to Lund and can be found elsewhere (for example, at the Ullevål Hospital in Oslo, Norway; see *Dagens nyheter,* September 16, 1999). There are several variants on the same theme, for example, MORS MAGISTER VITAE, "Death is the teacher of life" (Broberg, 69). Since 1997, this building has housed the Department of Cultural Science, jokingly referred to as "the department of cultural anatomy." *Kulturanatomiska studier* describes several interesting aspects of the activities of anatomists at the University of Lund from the perspective of the history of ideas. On the building's design, see Hjördis Kristensson, *Vetenskapens byggnader under 1800-talet: Lund och Europa* (Lund: Arkitekturmuseum, 1990), 266–69.

2. *Kroppen efter döden: Slutbetänkande av transplantationsutredningen* (Stockholm: Allmänna förlaget, 1992), 101, 233; hereafter referred to as SOU (Statens Offentliga Utredningar) 1992:16.

3. In Swedish medical contexts, the term *dissektion* (dissection) was still used into the 1900s, interchangeable with the term *sektion.* The term *liköppning* (the opening of a corpse) was also used, but it had the disadvantage of being less precise; it can be applied to any dissection, as well as to clinical and forensic autopsies.

4. See Foucault, *Birth of the Clinic.*

5. The history of the anatomical sciences in Sweden is described in Carl Gustaf Ahlström, "Arvid Florman—den förste patologen i Lund," in *Sydsvenska medicinhistoriska sällskapets årsskrift* Lund, 1975); also by the same author, "Ett gammalt museum berättar: Glimtar från patalogiska institutionens museum i Lund," in *Sydsvenska medicinhistoriska sällskapets årsskrift* (Lund, 1982); and "Patologisk anatomi i Lund 1668–1962," in *Sydsvenska medicinhistoriska sällskapets årsskrift,* supplementum 2 (Lund, 1983); Telemak Fredbärj, "De offentliga anatomierna i Sverige under 1600-och 1700-talen," in *Medicinhistorisk årsbok 1958* (Stockholm, 1958); Gustafsson, *Själens biologi;* Johannisson, *Kroppens tunna skal.* On the history of the Karolinska Institute, see *Karolinska mediko-kirurgiska institutets historia,* vols. 1–3 (Stockholm, 1910), hereafter cited as *KI's historia;* Julius Rocca, *Forging a Medical University: The Establishment of Sweden's Karolinska Institutet* (Stockholm: Karolinska Institutet University Press, 2006). See also the forthcoming edited volume on the history of the Karolinska Institute, which will be published in conjunction with the institute's bicentenary in 2010 (eds. Karin Johannisson, Ingemar Nilsson, and Roger Qvarsell). On the conflicts between

the Karolinska Institute and the two older medical faculties, see especially Sven-Eric Liedman, *Israel Hwasser* (Uppsala: Uppsala universitet, 1971); Ulf Lagerkvist, *Karolinska institutet och kampen mot universiteten* (Hedemora, Sweden: Gidlunds, 1999).

6. Erik Müller, "Anatomiska institutionen," *KI's historia*, vol. 3, 69.

7. According to ibid., 121, of the 20 to 30 anatomy students at the Karolinska Institute in the 1840s and the 50 to 60 students in the 1850s, most were from the universities. The highest number of "dissectors" at the Karolinska Institute was enrolled during the 1880s—138 students per semester. After this, the number decreased (ibid., 125, 135). The reason the numbers varied so greatly is unclear.

8. Magnus Huss, *Några skizzer och tidsbilder från min lefnad: Hämtade dels från äldre anteckningar, dels ur minnet vid 78 års ålder* (Stockholm: Norstedt, 1891), 11. The body parts being dissected were called "portions" and were often chosen according to a certain system, for example, the muscles and ligaments of the arm or the nerves of the face.

9. *KI's historia*, vol. 1, 281–83.

10. Huss, *Några skizzer* 38.

11. Kristenson, *Vetenskapens byggnader,* 45.

12. Weimarck Akademi och anatomi, 197–98. See also Axel Key, *Till kirurgins historia i Sverige* Stockholm, 1897), 95; Müller, "Anatomiska institutionen," 74; Fredbärj, "De offentiga anatomierna," 15.

13. Edvard Clason, *Ordningsreglor för arbetet vid anatomiska institutionen.* "Huru bör man dissekera? Föreläsning vid öppnandet af den nya dissektionssalen d. 10 Nov. 1884" (Uppsala, 1885) 2.

14. Israel Holmgren, *Mitt liv*, vol. I (Stockholm: Natur och kultur, 1959), 49. Holmgren describes his "life in the anatomy hall" as "very pleasant" and "happy," despite Professor Clason's originality and the lack of hygiene, even squalor (50–51).

15. Another picture of a corpse cellar exists in Gaston Backman's photo album in the Uppsala University library's Maps and Prints department. This picture seems to have been taken to show a device used to lift bodies out of tubs of preservatives. This lifting device looks like a large metal claw; loaded with a dead body, it is reminiscent of old torture devices. Despite this, the men in the picture look content, making the picture even more gruesome. Conditions and practices were very similar in Denmark and Sweden at the time, making the Danish photograph representative.

16. For a history of forensic medicine in Sweden, see Tony Gustafsson, *Läkaren, döden och brottet: Studier i den svenska rättsmedicinens etablering* (Uppsala: Acta Universitatis Upsaliensis, 2007).

17. Algot Key-Åberg, "Gällande bestämmelser rörande tillgången till lik för den antomiska undervisningen i Stockholm, Upsala och Lund," *Hygiea* (1889), 1–2. Regarding illegitimate children, this text delineates "all of the illegitimate children who are either murdered or who die," indicating that it is a question of newborn children; however, age is not clearly specified. The rules concerning anatomy are somewhat different for Stockholm and the university towns. However, the differences are small and would take up too much space to discuss here; further, doing so would not be useful, since my focus is on attitudes. I will not always note the different towns the rules cover. The rules are also often convoluted and difficult to understand. I have placed greater emphasis on making my presentation comprehendible and suited to the context than on reproducing the rules exactly. For the early history of anatomy

in Sweden, see Fredbärj, *De offentliga anatomierna;* Weimarck, *Akademi och anatomi;* Vilhelm Djurberg, *När det var anatomisal på Södermalms stadshus i Stockholm 1685–1748* (Stockholm: Norstedts, 1927). Turku is now situated in Finland, which was part of Sweden until 1809.

18. Key-Åberg, *Gällande bestämmelser,* 6.

19. Ibid., 7–9.

20. Ibid., 6–7.

21. Ibid., 19. This regulation concerned transport from prisons.

22. *KI's historia* reports the economic situations of the various institutions, including donations and government contributions (those applied for, those granted, and those refused). See, for example, vol. 1, 261–62.

23. I have examined collections of regulations regarding the medical system between 1860 and 1932 with respect to everything involving the handling of dead bodies. In many cases the legal texts are difficult to interpret. To obtain the best result, it would be necessary to also examine the proposals and reports that led to the formulation of the laws, but such a task would constitute a separate study.

24. Stockholm provided the most corpses for anatomical uses of any place in Sweden. On April 26, 1861, the government legislated that "the institutions of medical education in Uppsala and Stockholm shall hereafter be given equal rights to thereby fill their needs for deceased bodies [that are] otherwise unmet in other locales." *Författningar m.m. angående medicinalväsendet i Sverige omfattande tiden från och med 1860 till och med år 1876, förra delen (1860–1873),* ed. A. Kullberg (Stockholm, 1877), 47.

25. At the same time, the military medical training program at Garrison Hospital in Stockholm submitted a request for more corpses for surgery practice. Key-Åberg, *Gällande bestämmelser,* 13; *Författningar m.m. angående medicinalväsendet i Sverige omfattande tiden från och med år 1877 till och med år 1882,* ed. D. M. Pontin (Stockholm, 1884), 174 (Kungliga Ecklesiastikdepartmentets skrifvelse d. 19 Nov. 1880 till Medicinalstyrelsen angående tillgång på menniskolik för den anatomiska undervisningen).

26. *Författningar . . . 1877 till och med år 1882,* 255 (Kungliga Ecklesiastikdepartmentets skrifvelse d. 26 Aug. 1881), (Kungliga Ecklesiastikdepartmentets embetsskrifvelse d. 7 December 1888); Key-Åberg, *Gällande bestämmelser,* 16.

27. *Samling af författningar och cirkulär m.m. angående medicinalväsendet,* serie A (Stockholm, 1926), 104.

28. Section 5, however, states that "the institution's chairman nonetheless has the right to consider whether bodies already sent to the institution may, due to special circumstances, and without scheduled dissection, be turned over for burial to persons as provided in §1 under (a) [that is, family members]." Sweden was governed by the Social Democratic Party from 1932 to 1976, as well as during part of the 1920s. Since the legislation presents a large degree of continuity over a long period, the laws do not reflect party politics in any straightforward manner.

29. It is unclear how the Royal Academy of Fine Arts used its ration of corpses. According to Torsten Weimarck, anatomical instruction held a central role even in the curriculums of the earliest fine arts academies. Anatomy continued in this role "in large part until the beginning of the 1900s, with a final high point at the end of the 1800's" (Weimarck, *Akademi och anatomi,* 8).

30. *Samling av författningar och cirkulär m.m. angående medicinalväsendet,* 65 (SFS 1932: 371).

31. Ibid. From 1949 on, this declaration also applied to corpses used for anatomical research (SOU 1992: 16, 75, 236).

32. SOU 1992: 16, 233.

33. Even more common, however, was the Swedish term *liköppning,* which means simply "the opening of a corpse." Today, the Swedish term for a clinical autopsy is *obduktion.*

34. SOU 1992: 16, 110.

35. Ibid.

36. Holmgren, *Mitt liv,* vol. 1, plate 21. Holmgren's caption does not indicate where the photograph was taken, but the autopsy table, lighting fixtures, and chairs match those in a photo from the Karolinska Institute's department of pathological anatomy in *KI's historia,* vol. 3, 370.

37. However, certain doctors argued in favor of the benefits of gloves, and new practices were about to be introduced. See Jacques Borelius, "Om aseptiska operationers utförande i sterila bomullsvantar samt septiska operationers och obduktioners utförande i gummihandskar," *Hygiea* 2 (1898).

38. For example, Gustaf Retzius was autopsied in his bedroom, after which his brain was preserved using his own method of curing in formalin and was donated to the Karolinska Institute by his widow, Anna Hierta-Retzius. Gustafsson, *Själens biologi,* 139, 168. Gustafsson's source was Folke Henschen, *Min långa väg till Salamanca: En läkares liv* (Stockholm, 1957).

39. *Förhandlingar vid Svenska Läkare-Sällskapets Sammankomster 1874* (Stockholm, 1874), 101. In *Att leva som lytt: Handikappades levnadsvillkor i 1800-talets Linköping* (Linköping, 1999), Ingrid Olsson discussed a similar case described by Sven Hedin in the early nineteenth century," En händelse af en Hydrocephalus internus beskrifven," *Kongl. Vetenskapsakademiens Nya Handlingar* [Stockholm, 1807], 69–71).

40. *Förhandlingar vid Svenska Läkare-Sällskapets Sammankomster1893* (1894), 222.

41. Cited in connection with the April 26, 1861, regulation, in *Författningar . . . 1860 till och med år 1876,* 47. Italics are mine.

42. Ibid.

43. Ibid., 509.

44. Ibid., 512–13.

45. *K.Maj:ts nådiga lasarettsstadga d. 18 okt 1901* (Stockholm, 1901), ch. 3, §28:12. Italics are mine.

46. SOU 1992: 16, 129. The 1992 commission on legislation for organ procurement and transplants maintained: "According to the proposition [for the 1976 law], consideration for the dignity of the deceased and for his family led to the prescription of such a responsibility. It was furthermore felt that the ruling contained the advantage of bringing legislation into better agreement with corresponding laws in Denmark and Norway."

47. Algot Key-Åberg, *För obduktionsbordet: Författningar och protokoll jämte utlåtanden* (Stockholm, 1916), 73–174.

48. Ibid., 79.

49. Eduard Ritter von Hofmann, *Rättsmedicinsk atlas* (Stockholm, 1898). Translation from the original German version, *Atlas der gerichtlichen Medizin* (München: Lehmann, 1889).

50. Jordanova, *Sexual Visions;* Ulrika Nilsson, "Att ta till kniven," in *Det givna och det föränderliga: En antologi om biologi, människobild och samhälle,* ed. Nils Uddenberg (Nora, Sweden: Nya Doxa, 2000).

51. For a detailed history of forensic medicine in Sweden, see Gustafsson, *Läkaren, döden och brottet.*

52. SOU 1992: 16, 76.

53. *Författningar . . . år 1886,* ed. D. M. Pontin (Stockholm, 1887), 4–7.

54. Ibid., 7–15. This regulation required 7½ pages, as opposed to 2½ pages for the previous one.

55. Johan Petrus Norberg, *"Norbergska målet": Medicinskt rättsfall i Gefle 1896* (Gävle, Sweden, 1897), 4.

56. Ibid., 7–9; *Handlingar rörande Norbergska målet, del. I: Rättegångshandlingar från rådhusrätten i Gefle* (Lund, 1897), 14, 32, 61, 67, 69.

57. *Handlingar rörande Norbergska målet I,* 111.

58. Norberg, *"Norbergska målet,"* 9.

59. Richardson, *Death, Dissection, and the Destitute,* 30–31. For conditions in the United States, see Sappol, *Traffic of Dead Bodies,* chapter 4.

60. Åkesson, *Mellan levande och döda,* 41–42. Åkesson's argument deals with forensic pathologists, but it can be extended to doctors in general. In the late 1800s it was obvious, even to the doctors themselves, that discrepancies existed between the ways doctors and the general public regarded dead bodies. For example, Edvard Clason mentioned this point in a discussion of how students acquire a professional attitude (*Huru bör man dissekera*). See the discussion of the beneficial and the grotesque body later in this chapter.

61. Gunnel Hedberg, "Straffet offentligen ske på hans bild och efterliknelse: Några anteckningar till ett lagförslag 1696 om införande av avrättning in effigie i Sverige," *RIG: Kulturhistorisk tidskrift grundad 1918* 1 (1998): 20. SOU 1992: 16, addendum B, contains a summary of the positions of various religions regarding anatomy and autopsy.

62. Hagberg, *När döden gästar,* esp. chapter 31.

63. Ibid., chapter 2.

64. On executions, see Richard J. Evans, *Rituals of Retribution: Capital Punishment in Germany 1600–1987* (Oxford: Oxford University Press, 1996); V.A.C. Gatrell, *The Hanging Tree: Execution and the English People, 1770–1868* (Oxford: Oxford University Press, 1994); Martin Monestier, *Peines de mort: Histoires et techniques des exécutions capitales des origines à nos jours* (Paris: Le Cherche Midi Editeur, 1994).

65. Torbjörn Gustafsson, "Frithiof Holmgren och straffanatomin," *Tvärsnitt* 2 (1995): 36.

66. See, for example, Johannisson, *Kroppens tunna skal,* 42.

67. Hedberg, "Straffet offentligen ske . . . ,." The custom of punishing a surrogate body survives today and can be seen primarily in protest demonstrations, which may include the execution of an effigy or a symbolic funeral procession.

68. Quoted in Key-Åberg, *Gällande bestämmelser,* 8.

69. Quoted in ibid.

70. See Richardson, *Death, Dissection, and the Destitute,* chapter 2.

71. Göran Inger, "Rätten över eget liv och över egen kropp," in *Kungl. Humanistiska Vetenskaps-Samfundet i Uppsala: Årsbok 1985* (Uppsala: Uppsala universitet, 1986), 95.

72. SOU 1992: 16, 236.

73. Johannisson, *Kroppens tunna skal,* 40–42.

74. Gustafsson, *Själens biologi,* 167–69.

75. Richardson, *Death, Dissection, and the Destitute,* 159–60.

76. Erik Müller, "Några ord om anatomien såsom vetenskap och läroämne" (inaugural lecture, Karolinska Institute, September 8, 1899), *Hygiea* 2 (1899): 491.

77. Ibid., 497–99.

78. Clason, "Huru bör man dissekera," 12.

79. Ibid., 11–12. Clason's praise of purity stands in complete opposition to the image of the squalid anatomy halls in his day, as described by Israel Holmgren. Among other things, Clason is said to have handled corpses during the exercises (without gloves) and immediately thereafter to have run his fingers through his beard (Holmgren, *Mitt liv,* vol. 1, 50).

80. Compare the ideal of objectivity posited by physiologist Claude Bernard with his much-criticized attitude toward vivisections (experiments on living animals): "The physiologist is no common human being; he is a learned man who is possessed and absorbed by the scientific idea he pursues. He does not hear the cries of the animals, he no longer sees the blood flowing, he sees only his idea and understands only the organisms which conceal from him the problems he seeks to solve" (quoted in Gustafsson, *Själens biologi,* 70).

81. Clason, "Huru bör man dissekera," 10–11.

82. Swedish folklorist Bengt af Klintberg presents two such stories in his work on urban legends, *Råttan i pizzan: Folksägner i vår tid* (Stockholm: Norstedts, 1986), nos. 79 and 80 (214–17).

83. John Harley Warner and James M. Edmonson, *Dissection: Photographs of a Rite of Passage in American Medicine, 1880–1930* (New York: Blast Books, 2009); Sappol, *Traffic of Dead Bodies,* chapter 3.

84. Bachtin quoted in Katharine Young, *Presence in the Flesh: The Body in Medicine* (Cambridge, MA: Harvard University Press, 1997), 108.

85. Ibid., 110.

86. Ibid., 119.

87. Ibid., 128–29.

88. Examples of such pictures have been published in Gustafsson, "Frithiof Holmgren," 33; *Kulturanatomiska studier,* 75.

89. Martin Kemp and Marina Wallace, *Spectacular Bodies: The Art and Science of the Human Body from Leonardo to Now* (Berkeley and London: University of California Press and Hayward Gallery, 2000); John Harley Warner and Lawrence J. Rizzolo, "Anatomical Instruction and Training for Professionalism from the 19th to the 21st Centuries," *Clinical Anatomy* 19 (2006).

90. Motzi Eklöf, *Läkarens ethos: Studier i den svenska läkarkårens identiteter, intressen och ideal 1890–1960* (Linköping, 2000), chapter 4: On the concept of homosociality, see Eve Kosofsky Sedgwick, *Between Men: English Literature and Male Homosocial Desire* (New York: Columbia University Press, 1985).

91. Israel Holmgren, in his memoirs, maintained that this was one of Clason's "favorite themes" and that "using anatomical structures as his point of departure, [he] loved to enter into social considerations" (Holmgren, *Mitt liv,* vol. 1, 50).

92. On the attitudes of early female and male doctors on this topic, see Ulrika Nilsson, *Kampen om Kvinnan: Professionalisering och konstruktioner av kön i svensk gynekologi*

1860–1925 (Uppsala: Acta Universitatis Upsaliensis, 2003); Nilsson, "Kön, klass, och vetenskaplig auktoritet: Om kvinnliga läkarpionjärer," in *Vetenskapsbärarna: Naturvetenskapen i det svenska samhället 1880–1950*, ed. Sven Widmalm (Hedemora, Sweden: Gidlunds, 1999); Ulrika Nilsson and Kristina Eriksson, "Kön och professionalisering: Om kvinnliga och manliga läkares strategier 1900 och 2000," in *Idéhistoriska perspektiv: Symposium i Göteborg, Arachne* 16 (Göteborg, 2000); Eklöf, *Läkarens ethos*, chapter 4.

93.   Carl Sundberg, "Patologisk-anatomiska institutionen," in *KI's historia*, vol. 3 (Stockholm, 1910), 363. The assistant was Anna Strecksén, Sweden's first female medical doctor, who received her doctoral degree for a dissertation on the pathogenesis of cancer. Strecksén died at only thirty-four as a result of poisoning, which she probably acquired through her laboratory work. See Nilsson, "Kön, klass, och vetenskaplig auktoritet," 177, note 13.

94.   Holmgren *Mitt liv*, vol. 1, 128. In her books *Den mörka kontinenten* and *Kroppens tunna skal*, Karin Johannisson described the development of scientific subordination.

95.   Bodil Persson, *När kvinnorna kom in i männens värld: Framväxten av ett kvinnligt tekniskt yrke—laboratorieassistent under perioden 1880–1941* (Malmö, 1994), quotation on 184. See also Ulla Wikander, *Delat arbete, delad makt; om kvinnans underordning i och genom arbetet: En historisk essä* (Uppsala: Institutionen för ekonomisk historia, Uppsala universitet, 1991).

96.   Cynthia Eagle Russett, *Sexual Science: The Victorian Construction of Womanhood* (Cambridge, MA: Harvard University Press, 1989); Londa Schiebinger, *Nature's Body: Gender in the Making of Modern Science* (Boston: Beacon, 1993); Maja Larsson, *Den moraliska kroppen: Tolkningar av kön och individualitet i 1800-talets populärmedicin* (Hedemora, Sweden: Gidlund, 2002).

97.   Gustafsson, *Själens biologi*, 174. Within medical science, an internal debate raged over which facts provided justification for the subordinate ranking of women and "the lower races." Gustaf Retzius, for example, felt it was impossible in an absolute sense to link lower brain weight or less complex convolutions to a lower level of intelligence. The fact that persons possessing such traits were more poorly equipped than white males, however, seems to have been self-evident. Gustafsson shows that despite his determined attempts, Retzius could not prove that decisive differences existed between the brains of people of various races: "This does not mean that Retzius took opposition to anthropologists' constant search for and claims of a racial hierarchy, or of differences between genders, races and social classes. Quite the opposite, it can be assumed that he shared these suppositions, but that he could not prove them scientifically" (190). Chapter 3, "Anthropologists and Morality," in Gustafsson addresses the problem of mathematician Sonja Kovalevsky's brain. Also see Hertha Hansson, *Alkemi, romantik och rasvetenskap: Om en vetenskaplig tradition* (Nora, Sweden: Nya Doxa, 1994).

98.   Sappol, *Traffic of Dead Bodies*, 81.

99.   See, for example, Bringéus, "Vår hållning till döden, speglad," *Svensk begravningssed, Livets högtider*, "Vår hålling till döden"; Walter, *Revival of Death*. Doctors, especially physiologists, devoted themselves to understanding death and its effects on the systems of the body. A study of this discourse concerning death would be of interest, but it cannot be made here. See Hans Bendz, *Bidrag till kännedomen om hängningsdödens fenomen, Lunds universitets årsskrift* 21 (Lund, 1885); Hilding Bergstrand,

Till frågan om vad som bör innefattas i begreppet mänskligt liv i rättslig mening (Stockholm, 1916); Frithiof Holmgren, *Om halshuggning betraktad från fysiologisk synpunkt* (Uppsala, 1876); Einar Sjövall, *Om döden: En biologisk överblick* (Lund, 1915); Hjalmar Öhrvall, *Den fysiologiska döden och dess betydelse för lifvet* (Stockholm, 1899).

100. On the development of a nomenclature of death, see Lennart Nordenfelt, *Causes of Death—A Philosophical Essay* (Stockholm: FRN, 1983).

Chapter Three

1. The departments of anatomy, pathology, and histology each had museum collections. See the articles on each department in *KI's historia*, vol. 3.

2. In 1999, Lütze's wax museum was shown at the Museum of National Antiquities in Stockholm. See the exhibition catalog, *Ett resande vaxkabinett*, ed. Inga Lundström and Katarina Svensson (Stockholm: Statens historiska museum, 1999). The owner of this wax museum is Per Simon Edström, who wrote *Mördaren och helvetesmaskinen: En egensinnig anteckningsbok om en flerårig detektivundersökning av ett resande vaxkabinett och vaxkabinetten i Norden* (Värmdö, Sweden: Arena Theatre Institute, 2005)

3. For the history of popular anatomy shows in America, see Sappol, *Traffic of Dead Bodies*, chapter 9.

4. If no other source is indicated, information about the facilities, meetings, and other aspects of the Swedish Society of Medicine is taken from Frithiof Lennmalm's history of the society, *Svenska Läkaresällskapets historia 1808–1908* (Stockholm: Svenska Läkaresällskapet, 1908). The society's regular meeting time was seven o'clock on Tuesday evenings, and more than 125 doctors often attended the meetings during the 1890s (Lennmalm, 393).

5. Ibid., chapters 9 and 10. See also Gunnar Nilsson, *Svenska Läkaresällskapets historia 1908–1938* (Stockholm: Svenska Generalstabens litografiska anstalts förlag, 1947).

6. Lennmalm's second addendum lists everything the society published from 1808 to 1908. It shows that in addition to a number of festschrifts, occasional papers, special announcements, cholera reports, and similar documents, the society also published membership lists, its regulations, and *Sveriges Läkarehistoria (The History of Physicians in Sweden)*. After 1864, *Svenska Läkaresällskapets Handlingar* was renamed *Svenska Läkaresällskapets Nya Handlingar.*

7. See, for example, Lennmalm, *Svenska Läkaresällskapets historia 1808–1908*, 357.

8. *Förhandlingar rid Svenska Läkaresällskapets Sammankomster* (1874), 100–103.

9. Lennmalm maintained "that a considerable portion of Key's pathological-anatomical scientific production was invested in these autopsy reports in *Läkaresällskapets Förhandlingar.* It is impossible here to mention even the most important of Key's works; it would be almost equal to making a register of all works on special pathological anatomy." Lennmalm, *Svenska Läkaresällskapets historia*, 356–57.

10. Judging from the scanty description, this fetus seems to have been fully developed, but it is unclear whether it was born dead, died during delivery, or died later. The same lack of clarity arises in many descriptions of deformed fetuses. This is

a result either of obvious points the doctors were able to interpret from the reports or the fact that information was deemed not of interest. Could it be that the attitude toward deformed fetuses was such that they were allowed to die, even when they might have had a chance to survive? The question would be an interesting one to research.

11. Lennmalm, *Svenska Läkaresällskapets historia* 275.

12. Especially prominent among Swedish researchers in teratology was Ivar Broman. His *Normale und abnorme Entwicklung des Menschen: Ein Hand- und Lehrbuch der Ontogenie und Teratologie, speziell für praktische Ärzte und Studierende der Medizin* (Wiesbaden, 1911) was used as a textbook on the subject. In the vein of popular science, Broman also published a rather terrifying book, *Vidunder och missfoster i fantasi och verklighet* (*Freaks and Monstrosities in Imagination and Reality*), as part of the popular science series *Bonniers små handböcker i vetenskapliga ämnen* (Stockholm: Bonniers, 1929).

13. See *KI's historia*, vol. 3, "Anatomiska institutionen" by Erik Müller, and "Patologisk-anatomiska institutionen" by Carl Sundberg. The departments' museum collections are discussed in more detail later in the chapter.

14. See Ulrik Quensel, "Om en ny metod att konservera anatomiska preparat med bibehållandet af de naturliga färgerna," *Hygiea* 9 (1897).

15. On the preservation of brains, see also Gustaf Retzius, "Om metoderna att konservera hjärnor," in *Biologiska föreningens förhandlingar*, vol. 1, no. 6 (Stockholm, 1889); Retzius, *Das Menschenhirn: Studien in der makroskopische Morphologie* (Stockholm, 1896); Ivar Broman, *Människohjärnan: En kortfattad handledning vid dess studium och dissektion* (Lund, 1926); Carl M. Fürst, "Professorn i Fysiologi vid Lunds universitet Magnus Blix' hjärna," in *Lunds universitets årsskrift*, part 2, vol. 14, no. 3 (Lund, 1918); Bror Gadelius, "Om förhållandet mellan psykiatri och hjärnanatomi: Installationsföreläsning hållen vid Karolinska Institutet den 16 mars 1904," Almänna Svenska Läkartidningen (Stockholm, 1904); Henschen, "Om den tekniska undersökningen af hjärnan."

16. Quotation from Gustaf Retzius lecture at Svenska Läkaresällskapet, April 24, 1894, in *Svenska Läkaresällskapets Förhandlingar* (1894) 157. "Macroscopic" refers to examinations that could be conducted without the use of a microscope. The implication here is that other characteristics are required of materials to be studied under the lens. Even the economic aspects of preparations are mentioned.

17. Cf. Sappol, *Traffic of Dead Bodies*, 2–3.

18. Emil Holmgren, *Lärobok i histologi* (Stockholm, 1920). Although the techniques were constantly being improved, certain basic methods had been developed in the nineteenth century. According to Holmgren, the paraffin cross-section method had been introduced in the 1860s (22).

19. Christian Lovén, "Om lymfvägarna i magsäckens slemhinna," in *Nordiskt medicinskt arkiv*, vol. 5, no. 26 (Stockholm, 1873). I have written about Lovén's article and its illustrations in "Visuella representationer av anatomins praktik och objekt: Fyra betraktelser," in *Mer än tusen ord: Bilden och de historiska vetenskaperna*, ed. Lars M. Andersson, Lars Berggren, and Ulf Zander (Lund: Historiska Media, 2001). Lovén was a protégé of Anders Retzius and later professor of physiology at the Karolinska Institute, but he did not limit himself strictly to physiology. The examination described in his article could more aptly be characterized as descriptive comparative

microscopic anatomy (or histology) rather than physiology, but it can also serve as an example of how impossible it was to separate one discipline from another at that point in time.

20. Lovén, "Om lymfvägarna i magsäckens slemhinna," 4–5.

21. On scientific drawings and photographs created at the Karolinska Institute, see Solveig Jülich, "Medicinen och fotografiets mekaniska objektivitet: Carl Cur-man och tillkomsten av Karolinska institutets fotografiska ateljé 1861," in *Lychnos* (Uppsala, 1998). It is evident that the cooperative work between artists and scientists did not always go so smoothly—for example, after conflicts with Björkman, Gustaf Retzius preferred to create his own illustrations. (Compare Gustaf Retzius, *Biografiska anteckningar och minnen*, vol. 2, ed. O. Walde [Uppsala 1933–48], 16.)

22. Gustaf Retzius, "Josef Hyrtl," *Hygiea* 2 (1894): 191–92.

23. Ibid., 192. Italics are mine. Regarding Hyrtl's preparations at the Karolinska Institute, see also Erik Müller, "Anatomiska institutionen," 130.

24. More of the senses than just sight are involved in this work, of course, as they are in medicine in general. On the role of the senses throughout medical history, see *Medicine and the Five Senses*, ed. W. F. Bynum and Roy Porter (Cambridge: Cambridge University Press, 1993).

25. On the use of photographic techniques in this context, see among others Jülich, "Medicinen och fotografiets mekaniska objektivitet"; *History of Photography* 3 (1999), on the theme of "Medicine and Photography."

26. See, however, Weimarck, *Akademi och anatomi*, which provides a quote from the late 1600s showing that within the artistic context there was a clear awareness of this problem (52). This awareness must certainly have existed among practitioners in other disciplines as well. On the other hand, the problem is seldom discussed in medical history studies on anatomical representations.

27. Ideas about seeing and images are also presented, for example, by Erik Müller in "Några ord om anatomin såsom vetenskap och läroämne." For a detailed analysis of techniques for making things visible in medicine based on a study of radiology, see Jülich, *Skuggor av sanning*.

28. Edvard Clason, "Huru bör man dissekera?" 2–3.

29. Ibid., 5.

30. Ibid., 2.

31. "Malheur à l'élève qui, nayant rien vu et ne voulant rien voir, tenterait de substituer une pâle immitation de la nature à la nature elle-même!" quoted in ibid., 6.

32. Ibid., 9.

33. Ibid., 6.

34. Ibid., 7.

35. Ibid., 8.

36. In Sweden, only a few wet preparations have been preserved, including some deformed fetuses in formalin. A few collections of bones have been preserved by the Museum of National Antiquities in Stockholm and the Osteological Section of the Department of Archaeology at Lund University. Gustaf Retzius's collection of craniums is preserved in Stockholm University's archaeo-osteological laboratory at Ulriksdal. Why anatomical collections have not been preserved in Sweden is an interesting question I hope to address in future research. In other places in Europe, such

as Paris and Bologna, similar collections have been preserved and are still exhibited with pride.

37. Müller, "Anatomiska institutionen," 129. I have used the anatomical museum at the Karolinska Institute as my example because Müller described it so well. The Department of Pathological Anatomy had its own separate museum, and several other departments had collections of preparations. See respective departmental histories in *KI's historia,* vol. 3.

38. Müller, "Anatomiska institutionen," 135, 131.

39. On physical anthropology and the history of racial thinking in Sweden, see Gunnar Broberg, "Lappkaravaner på villovägar," *Lychnos* (1981–82); Broberg, "Det antropologiska fotoalbumet," in *Mer än tusen ord: Bilden och de historiska vetenskaperna,* ed. Lars M. Andersson, Lars Berggren, and Ulf Zander (Lund: Nordic Academic Press, 2001); Jacob Christensson, "Sven Nilsson och Skandinaviens urinvånare," in *Kulturanatomiska studier, Ugglan* 15 (Lund, 2001); Gustafsson, *Själens biologi;* Hansson, *Alkemi, romantik och rasvetenskap;* Olof Ljungström, *Oscariansk antropologi: Etnografi, förhistoria och rasforskning under sent 1800-tal* (Hedemora: Gidlund, 2004).

40. Müller, "Anatomiska institutionen."

41. Ibid., 37.

42. On the relationship of anatomy and art up to the beginning of the nineteenth century, see Weimarck, *Akademi och anatomi;* Weimarck, *Den normala kroppen: Några förvandlingar i bildkonsten av ett anatomiskt motiv* (Stockholm: Symposion, 1989). See also Martin Kemp, "Medicine in View: Art and Visual Representation," in *Western Medicine: An Illustrated History,* ed. Irvine Loudon (Oxford: Oxford University Press, 1997); Kemp and Wallace, *Spectacular Bodies.*

43. Exhibition catalog by Gunvor Bonds, *Anatomier: Studieteckningar ur Konstakademiens samlingar* (Stockholm: Konstakademien, 1991), 6, 19–20.

44. The Academy of Fine Arts in Stockholm houses a painting by August Malmström from 1894, depicting Carl Curman instructing a class. Most of the students in the painting are women, but there are also three male students, which does not reflect the reality of anatomy classes: until 1903, men and women had separate classes (ibid., 35). The cover of *Lychnos* (1998) has a photograph of a similar scene, showing Curman surrounded by students.

45. Ibid., 6, 25.

46. Carl Larsson, from his autobiography *Jag* (1953), quoted in ibid., 6.

47. For the history of museum collections, see Tony Bennett, *The Birth of the Museum: History, Theory, Politics* (London: Routledge, 1995); Ludmilla Jordanova, "Objects of Knowledge: A Historical Perspective on Museums," in *The New Museology,* ed. Peter Vergo (London: Reaktion Books, 1989); Lorraine Daston and Katharine Park, *Wonders and the Order of Nature 1150–1750* (New York: Zone Books, 2001); Gunnar Broberg and Sverker Sörlin, "Umgänget med muserna," *Tvärsnitt* 1–2 (1991). There is now a vast literature on this topic, which is a growing field of academic inquiry.

48. Eva-Lena Karlsson, KAT. NR. 313, *Ansikte mot ansikte: Porträtt från fem sekel,* ed. Görel Cavalli Björkman (Stockholm: Nationalmuseum/Atlantis, 2001), 255. A wax sculpture of Bébé, whose real name was Nicholas Ferry, is also kept in Paris in the large anatomical and pathological museum Delmas-Orfila-Rouvière, which belongs to the medical department of the Université René Descartes, Paris V (see André Delmas,

"Le Musée Orfila et le Musée Rouvière," *Surgical and Radiological Anatomy: Journal of Clinical Anatomy* 17, supplement I [1995]: 293, plate S25).

49. Julius von Schlosser, "Geschicte der Porträtbildnerei in Wachs: Ein Versuch," in *Jarbuch der Kunsthistorische Sammlungen . . .* 29, no. 3 (Vienna, 1911); *Ansikte mot Ansikte,* 257.

50. *The Funeral Effigies of Westminster Abbey,* ed. Anthony Harvey and Richard Mortimer (Woodbridge, UK: Boydell, 1994).

51. David Freedberg, *The Power of Images: Studies in the History and Theory of Response* (Chicago: University of Chicago Press, 1989), chapter 9.

52. Among others, see Anna Katharina Märker, "Model Experts: The Production and Uses of Anatomical Models at La Specola, Florence, and the Josephinum, Vienna, 1775–1814" (unpublished Ph.D. dissertation, Ithaca, NY, Cornell University, 2005); *The Anatomical Waxes of La Specola,* ed. Joseph Renahan (Firenze: Arnaud, 1995); *Le Cere del Museo dell'Istituto Fiorentino di Anatomia Patalogica* (Firenze: Arnaud, [n.d.]).

53. Susan Leigh Star and James R. Griesemer, "Institutional Ecology, 'Translations' and Boundary Objects: Amateurs and Professionals in Berkeley's Museum of Vertebrate Zoology, 1907–1939," *Social Studies of Science* 19 (1989); Sappol, *Traffic of Dead Bodies,* chapter 9.

54. *A Guide to the Hunterian Museum: Bicentenary Edition* [Elizabeth Allen] (London: Royal College of Surgeons, 1993), 26. The core of the Hunterian Museum consists of the collections of the famous surgeon John Hunter (1728–93). The museum still exists, even though portions of the collection were destroyed in a German bombing raid during World War II. Many objects have been preserved, although the entire display has been reorganized.

55. See *Ett resande vaxkabinett;* Edström, *Mördaren och helvetesmaskinen.* For general information about wax museums in Sweden, see Gunnar Broberg, "Entrébiljett till en skandal," *Tvärsnitt* 1–2 (1991).

56. Anders Ekström, *Den utställda världen: Stockholmsutställningen 1897 och 1800-talets världsutställningar* (Uppsala: Nordiska museets förlag, 1994), 165, 168; *1897: Mediehistorier kring Stockholmsutställningen,* ed. Anders Ekström, Solveig Jülich, and Pelle Snickars (Stockholm: Statens ljud- och bildarkiv, 2006).

57. Johannesson, *Den massproducerade bilden,* 68–70. Johannesson also shows how this oil painting by Lindegren was popularized by being transferred to several media and distributed in huge quantities. First it was sold as a lithograph, then as a woodcut in the book, *Svenska målares taflor;* it then became a wax diorama and, as such, was represented in the illustrated weekly, *Ny Illustrerad Tidning* in 1878, when it was included in a collection of four dioramas depicting ethnic life at the World's Fair in Paris. See Lena Johannesson, "Pictures as News, News as Pictures: A Survey of Mass-Reproduced Images in 19th Century Sweden," in *Visual Paraphrases: Studies in Mass Media Imagery* (Uppsala: Uppsala Universitet, 1984), 32–33. Johannesson also dealt with the subject of wax figures in "Jo-Jon, David and Madame Tussaud: Notiser om franska revolutionens bildvärld," in *Mörkrum och transparens: Studier i europeisk bildkultur och i bildens historiska evidens* (Stockholm: Carlssons, 2001). See also Mark B. Sandberg, *Living Pictures, Missing Persons: Mannequins, Museums and Modernity* (Princeton: Princeton University Press, 2003).

58. *Svenska Panoptikons Vägvisare* (Stockholm, 1922), 13. More on the Svenska Panoptikon can be found in Broberg, "Entrébiljett till en skandal"; Hans Lepp,

"Svenska Panoptikon," in *Sankt Eriks Årsbok 1978* (Stockholm, 1978); Pelle Snickars, *Svensk film och tidig visuell masskultur 1900* (Stockholm: Aura förlag, 2001), 92–94; Staffan Tjerneld, *Stockholmsliv . . .*, vol. 1 (Stockholm: Norstedts, 1949), 159–65. On the Musée Grévin, see Vanessa R. Schwartz, *Spectacular Realities: Early Mass Culture in Fin-de-siècle Paris* (Berkeley: University of California Press, 1998).

59. Key was shown sitting in a group, together with director of national antiquities Hans Hildebrand and librarian Harald Wieselgren. *Vägvisare genom Svenska Panoptikon* (Stockholm, 1894), 26–28. Many of the scenes and figures from the 1890s remained in the museum until it closed. The scene showing the Lagerlunden café, however, had disappeared (*Svenska Panoptikons Vägvisare*, 1922). The Lagerlunden scene was also reproduced in Tjerneld, *Stockholmsliv*, vol. 1, 145.

60. The "Room of Death" (Dödsrummet), which contained approximately twenty-five death masks of famous persons, from kings to murderers, was originally located on the second floor but was later moved to the "Cellar of Terror" (*Vägvisare*, 1894, 922).

61. Regarding the marketing of wax museums, see my "Människokroppen som spektakel: Om vaxkabinett och deras marknadsföring kring sekelskiftet 1900," in *Reklam och hälsa: Levnadsideal, skönhet och hälsa i den svenska reklamens historia*, ed. Roger Qvarsell and Ulrika Torell (Stockholm: Carlsson, 2005). This study builds on an examination of the posters for wax museums in the poster collection of the Royal Library.

62. On the history of Madame Tussaud's, see Johannesson, *Mörkrum och transparens;* Schwartz, *Spectacular Realities; The Quick and the Dead: Artists and Anatomy*, ed. Deanna Petheridge and Ludmilla Jordanova (London: National Touring Exhibitions, 1997).

63. *Castans anatomiska museum: Katalog öfver Naturvetenskaplig-Anatomiska Afdelningen och Panoptikon-Afdelningen* (Örebro, Sweden, 1909), 2.

64. Ernst Almquist, "Hygieniska institutionen," in *KI's historia*, vol. 3. It is also unclear whether this was the same museum of hygiene that was put on display by the philanthropist Anna Hierta-Retzius at the 1897 Stockholm Exposition (Ekström, *Den utställda världen*, 179).

65. Roger Saban and Sylvie Hugues, "Les Musées d'Anatomie de l'Institut d'anatomie," *Histoire des Sciences Médicales* 33, no. 2 (1999): 175–76.

66. Ibid., 176.

67. Schwartz, *Spectacular Realities*, 97.

68. Jordanova, *Sexual Visions;* Johannisson, *Kroppens tunna skal;* Elisabeth Bronfen, *Over Her Dead Body: Death, Femininity and the Aesthetic* (Manchester: Manchester University Press, 1992); and Elaine Showalter, *Sexual Anarchy: Gender and Culture at the Fin-de-Siècle* (London: Bloomsbury, 1991) also consider the scientific anatomical waxes of women erotically inviting. It is true that certain characteristics are common among the wax figures most often used as examples, the eighteenth-century works in La Specola in Florence. The female waxes are whole-body figures and are shown lying on satin cushions and wearing necklaces; they also have real hair. Their skin is often intact except for the opened abdomen, and their hands rest in graceful positions. The body language and symbols exhibited by the male figures are different. Yet by the end of the nineteenth century, the differences in how the figures were shown in scientific displays were less obvious. The main difference between the later male

and female specimens was that the female ones depicted only the reproductive system, while the male specimens showed the entire human body. Certainly, this representation practice conveys power, violence, and conceptions of gender and sexuality, but it is rarely directly pornographic to the extent that it invites visual desire and enjoyment.

69. Schwartz, *Spectacular Realities*, 103.

70. Lepp, "Svenska Panoptikon," 165.

71. Jan Bondeson, "'Apkvinnan' Julia Pastrana," in *Medicinhistoriskt kuriosakabinett: Essayer* (Kivik, Sweden: Kiviksgårdens förlag, 1992), 255–81.

72. Pastrana's embalmed body has been exhibited in Sweden several times, including once in 1863 and most recently in 1973 (ibid., 274). Wax likenesses of Pastrana have been shown many times, including in 1895 in N. Nielsén's "Panoptikon och anatomiska museum," in which she was classified as a "phenomenon of nature" and described as an "ape woman from the Black Forest" (*Katalog N:o I öfver Patologiska afdelningen och Naturfenomenen* [Stockholm, 1863]); in 1909 in Castan's anatomical museum, in which she was called "the Bear Woman" (Castan's anatomiska museum, 5); and in 1914 in "Linu's internationella panoptikon," in which she was called "the human she-bear" (*Katalog öfver Linu's internationella panoptikon och anatomiska vaxmuseum* [Örebro, 1914], 4).

73. This poster is undated, but its text is largely identical to the text in an exhibition catalog, so the poster and catalog are presumably from the same establishment and time period. See *Katalog öfver Det stora Etnologiska, Geologiska, Anatomiska, Fysiologiska, Embryologiska och Patologiska Museum* (Stockholm, 1863), 20. According the catalog, she had performed in Stockholm with the Hinné and Renz circus. In the 1863 exhibition, both Pastrana's embalmed body and a wax figure of her were shown (6).

74. Cf. Harriet Ritvo, *The Platypus and the Mermaid, and Other Figments of the Classifying Imagination* (Cambridge, MA: Harvard University Press, 1997), chapter 4, "Out of Bonds."

75. Cf. Rebecka Lennartsson, *Malaria urbana—Om byråflickan Anna Johannesdotter och prostitutionen i Stockholm kring 1900* (Stockholm, 2001), 79–81. Lennartsson even characterizes prostituted women as objects in the voyeuristic culture of the turn of the twentieth century, in which they functioned as representatives "of the frightening and alluring Other: through her gender, often through her class status, and through her association with the city's dangerous dark side."

76. For a similar discussion of the phenomenon of the freak show and its cultural meanings, see Rosemarie Garland Thomson, *Extraordinary Bodies: Figuring Physical Disability in American Culture and Literature* (New York: Columbia University Press, 1997), 63–66. For further reading on the cultural construction of freaks, see Robert Bogdan, *Freak Show: Presenting Human Oddities for Amusement and Profit* (Chicago: University of Chicago Press, 1988).

77. See Star and Griesemer, "Institutional Ecology."

78. Thomson has also dealt with this topic; see, for example, *Extraordinary Bodies*, 76.

79. Ibid., chapter 3; Bogdan, *Freak Show*, 230.

80. Thomson, *Extraordinary Bodies*, 70.

81. Ibid., 74. See also Bogdan, *Freak Show*.

82. Thomson, *Extraordinary Bodies*, 79.

83. See Schwartz, *Spectacular Realities;* Snickars, Svensk film; Jülich, *Skuggor av sanning;* Anders Ekström, "Konsten att se ett landskapspanorama: Om åskådningspedagogik och exemplarisk realism under 1800-talet," in *Publika kulturer: Att tilltala allmänheten 1700–1900: En inledning* (Uppsala: Institutionen för idé- och lärdomshistoria, Uppsala universitet, 2000); Per-Markku Ristilammi, "Optiska illusioner—fetischism mellan modernitet och primitivism," *Kulturella perspektiv* 3 (1995); Ristilammi, "The Bodily Eye: Reflections on the Era of the Stereoscope," in *Amalgamations: Fusing Technology and Culture,* ed. Susanne Lundin and Lynn Åkesson (Lund: Nordic Academic Press, 1999).

84. Schwartz, *Spectacular Realities,* chapters 3–5.

85. Ludmilla Jordanova, "Museums: Representing the Real?" *Realism and Representation: Essays on the Problem of Realism in Relation to Science, Literature, and Culture,* ed. George Levine (Madison: University of Wisconsin Press, 1993), treats realism, representation, power, and order in relation to scientific and medical museums. The study uses the concrete examples of historical museums such as the Hunterian Museum and also examines the extreme form of realism presented in wax figures, the cult of genuinity, and similar phenomena. However, following Jordanova's reasoning at length would lead away from this study's focus on death.

86. Broberg, "Entrébiljett till en skandal," 124. See also Tony Bennett, "Pedagogic Objects, Clean Eyes, and Popular Instructions: On Sensory Regimes and Museum Didactics," *Configurations: A Journal of Literature, Science, and Technology* 6, no. 3 (1998).

87. Broberg, "Entrébiljett till en skandal," 120; Retzius, "Josef Hyrtl," 192.

88. Jordanova, "Museums," 255.

89. Johannisson, *Kroppens tunna skal,* 48–49. The chapter from which this quotation is taken, "Den anatomiska teatern," has been an important source of inspiration for me.

90. For a similar presentation, see Star and Griesemer, "Institutional Ecology."

Chapter Four

1. Verdier, *Façons de dire, façons de faire.* Here I refer to the Swedish edition, *Tvätterskan, kokerskan, sömmerskan: Livet i en fransk by genom tre kvinnoyrken* (Stockholm: Atlantis, 1981), 95, 113. Other women, either neighbors or relatives, might assist at a birth or a death. However, the person who became a help-wife always had both of these jobs in her repertoire. In addition, she held an especially high position in the village and enjoyed great respect (120).

2. Ibid., 113–15.

3. Ibid., 115–17.

4. See the discussion of the dangerous body in chapter 1.

5. Verdier, *Tvätterskan, kokerskan, sömmerskan,* 117–18 (quotation on 118).

6. Ibid., 118–19.

7. For a critical discusion of Swedish ethnology of the early 1900s, see Lilja, *Föreställningen om den ideala uppteckningen.*

8. Here, primarily the archives of N. E. Hammarstedt and the Etnologiska undersökningen (*Folkminnessamlingen: Död och begravning*) were used. The reports in

the Etnologiska undersökningen (EU) were recorded in the 1940s. The later reports tell stories from the late nineteenth and early twentieth centuries, while the older reports deal with earlier eras. The material varies in nature, reflecting shifting ethnological theories and methods. The material from the early 1900s focuses on the generalistic and the ancient and uses phrases such as "it was customary to," "in the area," and "in this region," while the material from the postwar years and later seeks more and more obviously to record personal, specific, and time-specific experiences from the informants' memories. Cf. ibid. References to material in the archives of the Nordic Museum use the abbreviation EU, plus the number of the individual record or excerpt. Only a few records from the *Kulturhistoriska undersökningen* (KU) have been used.

9. EU 52710 from Värmland. The informant was a woman born in 1888.

10. Ulrika Wolf-Knuts, "Liktvättning—ett kvinnoarbete," in *Budkavlen* (Åbo: Åbo Akademi, 1983).

11. Hagberg, *När döden gästar,* 127–28.

12. KU 3179.

13. Reply to questionnaire no. 39, "Man och kvinna," for example, EU 2714, 2739, 3044, 3064, 3238, 3639.

14. EU 31332.

15. Hagberg, *När döden gästar,* 128; EU 26801 from Västergötland; EU 7129.

16. EU 54643.

17. Hagberg, *När döden gästar,* 130–32; Verdier, *Tvätterskan, kokerskan, sömmerskan,* 113; EU 18147, 5678.

18. EU 24073.

19. Hagberg, *När döden gästar,* 227–29, chapter 13.

20. In Sweden today it is less common to display the deceased. If the family sees the dead body at all, it is often in a bed at a health care facility, although it may also be in a casket in an out-of-the-way room. If no one sees the corpse, its clothing serves a different function than is the case if it is viewed by a large number of funeral guests. On the role played by funeral home directors in leading rites, see Bremborg, "Från stigmatisering till professionalisering?" 58–64; Bremborg, "Yrke: begravningsentreprenör."

21. Among others, see EU 28605 from Bohuslän and 4122 from Småland. The details in this section are also verified by Hagberg, *När döden gästar,* chapter 7, "Den sista vilobädden."

22. See esp. EU 3108 from Bohuslän.

23. See esp. EU 31138 from Bohuslän and EU 23960 from Värmland.

24. See esp. EU 23511 from Bohuslän and EU 23331 from Södermanland.

25. See esp. EU 21446, 21310. These examples are from Dalarna, but similar reports exist from other portions of the country.

26. EU 42815.

27. EU 54641 from Härjedalen.

28. Unnumbered report in the Nordic Museum Archives (NMA), *Folkminnessamlingen: Död och begravning,* vol. 1, recorded by Brynhild Wilén in 1928.

29. See esp. EU 23405 from Småland and 31031 from Uppland.

30. Hagberg, *När döden gästar,* 194–95.

31. EU 8154.

32. EU 51993.
33. Hagberg, *När döden gästar,* 180.
34. Ibid., 125. Hagberg took this report from G. O. Hyltén-Cavallius, *Wärend och Wirdarne: Ett försök i svensk etnologi* (Stockholm, 1863–68).
35. EU 728.
36. EU 762. Both details are from Anna Arwidsson's reports.
37. EU 52338 from Skåne mentions that spruce, juniper, and boxwood would alleviate the smell of corpses.
38. Among others, see EU 728.
39. EU 31023 from Södermanland.
40. EU 52710 from Småland.
41. EU 9715. This report is a fascinating story on seventeen typewritten, folio-sized pages by S. af Ekström of Stockholm. The observations of this city dweller who had an interest in folk life convey an attitude that at once romanticizes and disparages the fisherfolk of the island of Rörö. The collisions of class and culture contained in the story are interesting and give evidence to the fact that different attitudes and ideas existed simultaneously and side by side.
42. Gary Laderman, *The Sacred Remains: American Attitudes toward Death, 1799–1883* (New Haven: Yale University Press, 1996). In the United States there are vocational courses in embalming and makeup techniques for corpses, as described in the novel *The Loved One: An Anglo-American Tragedy* by Evelyn Waugh (London: Penguin, 1951 [1948]). Regarding the funeral establishment in the United States, see also Gary Laderman, *Rest in Peace: A Cultural History of Death and the Funeral Home in Twentieth Century America* (Oxford: Oxford University Press, 2003); Metcalf and Huntington, *Celebrations of Death,* chapter 8; the classic *The American Way of Death* by Jessica Mitford (London: Hutchinson, 1963); and Mitford's follow-up book, *The American Way of Death Revisited* (New York: Alfred A. Knopf, 1998).
43. EU 52338. Funeral director Peggy Smith reported that her father, who returned to Sweden from the United States in 1909 and started a funeral home, introduced American-style caskets with glass in the lid. EU 54637.
44. EU 54643.
45. EU 54640.
46. EU 54641.
47. EU 54642.
48. EU 54639.
49. The history of funeral entrepreneurs given in this chapter is based on replies to the Nordic Museum's questionnaire no. 166, "Begravningsentreprenörsyrkets traditioner," as well as on reports taken by Ingrid Haraldson, a student, in the summer of 1957. Haraldson interviewed funeral home directors in Norrköping and Stockholm, and her results were used by Anna-Maja Nylén as supporting documentation for the formulation of questionnaire no. 166. When no reference is indicated in the text, the information has been extrapolated from several replies, as well as from reports in the NMA.
50. EU 31023.
51. EU 41248.
52. EU 48669.
53. KU 9.

54. EU 51993.

55. Ibid. Here the informant and the recorder were the same person, a farm wife born in 1889. Her report was made in 1961.

56. EU 56641.

57. EU 54637. It is unclear to what extent these firms dealt with anything above and beyond coffins. The informant wrote: "The word 'funeral director' (begravnings-entreprenör) did not exist then (around the turn of the century), and people said coffin shop, coffin factory or funeral home."

58. The general development sketched here is verified in both large and small details by Gabrielle Jeansson and Inga Kindblom, Kring livets högtider i Örkelljunga församling (Lund: Gleerup, 1968). The authors report that from the 1920s on, corpses were washed by the funeral home staff and that the washing of corpses had fallen out of practice by the 1930s. The first funeral home in Örkelljunga was established around 1918 (67–69). A mortuary was built in the 1930s, after which time the custom of saying farewell to the deceased in the home ceased (75). A similar development took place in the northern United States. Up until the Civil War, burial practices were managed by survivors with the assistance of undertakers and coffin makers. The funeral industry took a more organized form in the 1880s, starting in the growing urban centers of "modernizing America" (Laderman, Sacred Remains, 8–10, chapter 13). See also Laderman, Rest in Peace, especially chapter 1.

59. Sveriges Begravningsentreprenörers Förbund. Års-och Revisionsberättelse för år 1931: Protokoll över årsmötet den 17 juli 1932 [Stockholm], 1932.

60. For example, O. E. Arwidsson in Ingrid Haraldson's interview material, EU 54637.

61. SBF, constitution, 1932.

62. EU 54639.

63. EU 54637. Even today in Sweden, some funeral homes have deals with the police regarding the collection of deceased persons in cases of accidents, suicide, and similar types of deaths. See Åkesson, Mellan levande och döda, 75.

64. SBF, Års- och Revisionsberättelse för år 1931: Protokoll över årsmötet den 17 juli 1932 [Stockholm], 1932.

65. SBF, various meeting minutes and agreements, Swedish Royal Library, Ephemera.

66. The SBF was criticized harshly by organizations of the political left, and during the 1940s cooperative funeral associations were formed with the express purposes of making funerals and burial less expensive and breaking the funeral homes' monopoly. These associations were thus the predecessors to the contemporary Swedish cooperative funeral organization known as Fonus. See, for example, Viktor Petrén, "Reformerad begravningsverksamhet i Stockholm," in the journal of the Swedish cremation movement, Ignis 1 (1946); Lotte Mjöberg, Femtio år i livets tjänst: Fonus i dag, i går, i morgon (Stockholm: Informationsförlaget and Fonus, 1995).

67. EU 54637.

68. EU 54637.

69. SBF, Års- och Revisionsberättelse för år 1931.

70. Hagberg, När döden gästar, 197.

71. EU 54646.

72. EU 54637.

73.   Rudolf Broby-Johansen, *Dagens dont i Norden: Arbejdsbilledets historie i Danmark, Norge, Sverige, Finland, Island, på Färøerne, i Grønland og hos samerne* Aarhus: Fremad, 1972), 194.

74.   The title of the painting is *A Childhood Memory*. Broby-Johansen relates that Rissanen's father was carried home one winter evening after having frozen to death while fishing on the ice (ibid.). It is probably that childhood memory that is depicted in this painting.

75.   Among others, Arnold Karlsson and Anna Nilsson in Ingrid Haraldson's interview material, EU 54637.

76.   Lynn Åkesson, *Mellan levande och döda*, wrote that male dominance within the funeral industry in Sweden had begun to decrease during the last decades of the twentieth century (66).

77.   EU 54640.

78.   Anna Davidsson Bremborg, "Vem tar hand om den döda kroppen?" See also Bremborg, "Från stigmatisering till professionalisering?"

79.   A parallel historical development is illustrated by Sheila Adams in "A Gendered History of the Social Management of Death in Foleshill, Coventry, during the Interwar Years," in *The Sociology of Death: Theory, Culture, Practice,* ed. David Clark (Oxford: Blackwell, 1993). Compare also Lena Sommestad, *Från mejerska till mejerist: En studie av mejeriyrkets maskuliniseringsprocess* (Lund: Arkiv, 1992). I have borrowed the concept of the division of labor between the sexes from Sommestad.

80.   Wolf-Knuts, "Liktvättning," 72.

81.   In the old Swedish peasant culture, even washing the living body was mainly of a ritual nature and was not motivated by hygienic needs. Also, it was primarily visible parts of the body that were washed (Jonas Frykman and Orvar Löfgren, *Culture Builders: A Historical Anthropology of Middle Class Life* [New Brunswick: Rutgers University Press, 1987]. In this context, the authors refer to Marianne Eriksson, "Personlig hygien," in *Fataburen,* 1970).

82.   Wolf-Knuts, "Liktvättning," 64. The idea also occurs in Nils-Arvid Bringéus's writings on death and burial. See, for example, "Vår hållning till döden," 18.

83.   See, for example, EU 54640.

84.   Bringéus, *Klockringningsseden i Sverige.*

85.   Birgitta Skarin Frykman, "Det skulle visas utåt att man hade lik i huset . . ." in *Dödens riter,* ed. Kristina Söderpalm (Stockholm: Carlsson, 1994); Ingrid Nordström, "Begravningskalas," in the same book. Compare also the fear of dissection in the context of funerals of the poor, discussed in chapter 2. See also Richardson, *Death, Dissection, and the Destitute,* chapter 2. On the care of dead bodies among the English working class, see Adams, "Gendered History."

86.   EU 210. This example comes from Skåne. Not all informants were as class-conscious as this one, although class differences were less obvious in some parts of Sweden.

87.   Among others, see EU 210; KU 9.

88.   Compare Lilja, *Föreställningen om den ideala uppteckningen,* and Becker, "Picturing Our Past."

89.   Until 1926, when a new law came into effect, the Church of Sweden held the sole right to conduct funerals. This ruling was criticized by a number of groups, including the Free Churches, and beginning in 1910 the issue was debated in the

Swedish Parliament. See Pleijel, *Jordfästning i stillhet,* chapter 4. The fact that funerals within Free Church groups are not depicted in the NMA materials does not mean they did not occur. Pleijel wrote that Free Church preachers were able to conduct funerals according to their own rituals without risk of punishment. How this was achieved was described by Swedish Baptist leader Jacob Byström in a motion before the Swedish Parliament: when the grave had been filled back in, a narrow wooden chute that extended from the surface of the earth down to the lid of the coffin made it possible for a priest from the Church of Sweden to throw in three shovels of earth to complete the official church ritual (67–8).

90. Bringéus, "Vår hållning till döden."

91. The respondent wrote about "Greek-Catholic" funerals (it is unclear if he meant Catholic or Greek Orthodox funerals or if he was referring to Eastern Rite Catholics). O. E. Arvidsson, EU 54637, Ingrid Haraldson's interview material. Anna Wihlborg of Norrköping also mentioned that Jewish funerals featured a horse-drawn catafalque wagon, while at other funerals automobiles were used for transport.

92. EU 54639 mentions, for example, that money was put in both the coffin and the grave.

93. EU 54637.

94. EU 54643.

95. EU 54645. According to Angela Rundquist, *Blått blod och liljevita händer: En etnologisk studie av aristokratiska kvinnor 1850–1900* (Stockholm: Carlssons, 1989), 325, even at the highest levels of Swedish society, women were responsible for preparing dead bodies for burial.

Chapter Five

1. On the photo-historical context, see *Nouvelle Histoire de la Photographie,* ed. Michel Frizot (Paris: Bordas, 1994), as well as the Swedish photo history by Rolf Söderberg and Pär Rittsel, *Den svenska fotografins historia.* On page 136, Söderberg and Rittsel maintain that the easy-to-use cameras introduced in the 1880s made possible a new sort of amateur photography: photographing one's family for one's own album. In the beginning, however, this trend was limited to the more economically affluent levels of society. The responses to a questionnaire on portrait photography from the Nordic Museum Folklore Archive (no. 162 [1954]) indicate that amateur photography did not become widespread until the interwar years.

2. Similar photographs are preserved in other archives and collections, as well as in private homes. I have had no ambitions to make an inventory of these, and I have not conducted any systematic examination of the preserved collections of various photographers, in which one could undoubtedly find more material. Examples of Swedish photographic collections that include photographs of deceased persons include the Folklivsarkivet in Lund, the Minnesbank ("memory bank") at the Jämtland County Museum (see Britt Liljewall, *Självskrivna liv: Studier i äldre folkliga levnadsminnen* [Stockholm: Nordiska museets Forlag, 2001], 331), and the Thorin photographic collection in the Åtvidaberg Municipal Archives (thanks to Anita Andersson for this information).

3. Ruby, *Secure the Shadow*, 27.

4. Söderlind, *Porträttbruk i Sverige*, 152–56, 404–15; Sidén, *Den ideala barndomen*, chapter 5; Sidén, "Porträtt av döda," in *Ansikte mot ansikte: Porträtt från fem sekel*, ed. Görel Cavalli Björkman (Stockholm: Nationalmuseum/Atlantis, 2001), 155–61; *Naar het lijk: Het Nederlandse doodsportret 1500-heden*, ed. B. C. Sliggers (Haarlem, The Netherlands: Teylers Museum, 1998).

5. Söderlind, *Porträttbruk i Sverige*, figure 410; see also Söderlind, "Privat objekt och offentligt medium: Kungligt porträttbruk i Sverige—tidiga fotografiska bilder," in *Fotobilden: Historien i nuet—nuet i historien*, ed. Lena Johannesson, Angelika Sjölander-Hovorka, and Solfrid Söderlind (Linköping, Sweden: Linköpings universitet, 1989).

6. Hagberg uses different types of photographs of deceased persons at ten places in *När döden gästar*: 135, 185, 189, 193, 195, 197, 221, 223, 303, and 317.

7. See, for example, *Nouvelle Histoire de la Photographie*, 36; *Ljuva ögonblick—stunder av allvar*, ed. Tommy Arvidsson and Birgit Brånvall (Stockholm: Nordiska museet, 1994), 23; Russell Roberts, "Taxonomi: Om fotografins och klassificeringens historia," in *I skuggan av ljuset: Fotografi och systematik i konst, vetenskap och vardagsliv* (Stockholm: Moderna museet, 1998), 30; Rolf Söderberg, *Stockholmsgryning: En fotografisk vandring på Karl XV:s tid* (Stockholm: Liber, 1986), 86–88.

8. See Stanley Burns, *Sleeping Beauty: Memorial Photography in America* (New York: Twelvetrees, 1990); Hafsteinsson, "Post-mortem and Funeral Photography in Iceland"; Jensen, *Gennem lys og skygger;* Jensen, "Livet og døden i familiealbumet"; Bjarne Kildegaard, "Unlimited Memory: Photography and the Differentiation of Familiar Intimacy," in *Man and Picture: Papers from the First International Symposium for Ethnological Picture Research in Lund 1984*, ed. Nils-Arvid Bringéus (Stockholm: Almqvist and Wiksell International, 1986); Dan Meinwald, "Memento Mori: Death and Photography in Nineteenth Century America," text written for an exhibition at the California Museum of Photography in 1990, at http://vv.arts.ucla.edu/terminals/meinwald/meinwald.html (accessed May 20, 2009).

9. *Hvar 8 Dag* (June 16, 1901): 597–99.

10. Ibid., (September 22, 1901): 830.

11. Ibid., (August 25, 1901): 763; (September 1, 1901): 773, 778.

12. Ibid., (September 15, 22, and 29, 1907); (January 5, 1908). See Söderlind, *Porträttbruk i Sverige*, 411, for a comparison of pictures of and publications about the death and burial of King Oskar I.

13. *Hvar 8 Dag* 19, no. 2 (1901): 328.

14. Nationalmuseum NMH (Sweden's National Museum of Fine Arts drawing collection), 21, 1956.

15. Gustafsson, *Själens biologi*, 168.

16. Cf. EU 48135.

17. See Pleijel, *Jordfästning i stillhet*, on how the "silent funeral" (*begravning i stillhet*) became popular during the interwar years within wealthier circles, beginning in southern Sweden.

18. Hagberg, *När döden gästar*, 303. According to Hagberg, the photographer was N. P. Florén, and the photograph was taken in the 1890s. I have chosen to cite the information provided by the Nordic Museum.

19. Compare the discussion in Jan Garnert, "Rethinking Visual Representation: Notes on the Folklorist and Photographer Nils Keyland," *Nordisk Museologi* 2 (1995).

20. "Sam Lindskog, Kgl. Hoffotograf, Örebro," in *Från bergslag och bondebygd 1983,* ed. Egon Thun (Örebro, Sweden, Örebro läns hembygdsförbund and Stiftelsen Örebro läns museum, 1983), 9–11.

21. See Kildegaard, "Unlimited Memory."

22. From chapter 4 of this study, compare the section "Clothing the Deceased": clothing for deceased children was to be especially fancy.

23. Charlie E. Orr cited in Ruby, *Secure the Shadow,* 58.

24. In all likelihood, the reference here is to the Spanish flu, the severe influenza pandemic that swept through Europe in 1918–19. Cited in Clas Thor, *Ljusets hemligheter: Kvinnligt fotografi 1861–1986* (Örebro, Sweden: Morgonstjärnan, 1986), 36.

25. Liljewall, *Självskrivna liv,* 326, 331–33.

26. Ruby, *Secure the Shadow,* chapter 2, especially 76–78.

27. For example, EU 48104, 48106, 48113, 48127, 48128, 48131. The questions were primarily about the customs of earlier, rather than contemporary, times.

28. This interview was conducted by photography historian Anna Tellgren for her dissertation, published as *Tio fotografer: Självsyn och bildsyn: Svensk fotografi under 1950-talet i ett internationellt perspektiv* (Stockholm, Sweden, 1997). The interview is part of Tellgren's collection. (I thank Anna for allowing me access to it.)

29. The information obtained from these ten interviews cannot be taken as evidence that the same was true throughout Sweden and for all social and ethnic groups. To gain more complete knowledge of current conditions, a significantly larger number of interviews would have to be conducted, which has not been possible within the framework of this study. Nonetheless, the replies from these interviews are of value as an indication of something about which I would otherwise only have been able to speculate.

30. Karl-Erik O-n Ander, *Helsingborgs första fotografer och deras bilder 1840–1900* (Helsingborg, Sweden: K. E. O-n Ander, 1998), 14.

31. Ibid., 14.

32. See replies to questionnaire no. 162: notes in Folder 1, Nordic Museum, Folklore Archive.

33. Jensen, *Gennem lys og skygger;* Jensen, "Livet og døden i familiealbumet."

34. Jensen, "Livet og døden i familieabumet," 21–23.

35. EU 48135.

36. Compare Söderlind's reasoning concerning the death portrait photograph of Queen Desideria (Söderlind, *Portätlbruk i Sverige,* 415).

37. EU 48135.

38. See Jensen, "Livet og døden i familiealbumet," 30. Photographs of deceased children are, however, making a comeback and are recommended to parents as an aid in the grieving process (among others, see the same Jensen source, 22).

Chapter Six

Epigraph. Poem by Ernst Arendorff. These are the final lines of the poem Arendorff read at the founding of the local chapter of the Swedish Cremation Society in Kristinehamn, Sweden, in 1901. Arendorff was the chapter's secretary. The poem is from Oscar Övden, *Eldbegängelsens historia i Sverige 1882–1932* (Stockholm, 1932), 106.

1. *Eldbegängelsen—framtidens begravningsskick* (*Cremation—The Funeral Practice of the Future*) was the title of a small brochure by Oscar Övden, published by the Swedish Cremation Association as number 1 in its print series for 1929. Optimistic belief in progress and development was ever-present in the arguments presented by the cremation movement. I discuss the cremation movement in my *Renande lågor: Den svenska eldbegängelserörelsens framväxt under 1800-talets sista decennier* (Stockholm: Avdelningen för idéhistoria, Stockholms universitet, 1994), as well as in "Renande lågor: Om den svenska eldbegängelserörelsen kring sekelskiftet 1900," in *Från moderna helgonkulter till självmord: Föredrag från Idé- och vetenskapshistorisk konferens 1995*, ed. Thomas Kaiserfeld (Stockholm: Avdelningen för teknik-och vetenskapshistoria, KTH, 1995). The most complete study of the cremation movement in Sweden is a theological doctoral dissertation: Bengt Enström, *Kyrkan och eldbegängelserörelsen i Sverige 1882–1962* (Lund: Gleerup, 1964). See also Tuomo Lahtinen, *Kremering i Finland: Idéhistoria och utveckling* (Åbo: Åbo Akademi, 1989). Here I have avoided dwelling on the history of the cremation movement, as well as its relationship with the church and religion, since these aspects fall outside the scope of this study. For information on these subjects, refer to the studies cited in this note.

2. Carl Fehrman, *Kyrkogårdsromantik* (Lund: Gleerup, 1954); Göran Lindahl, *Grav och rum: Svenskt gravskick från medeltiden till 1800-talets slut* (Stockholm: Almqvist and Wiksell, 1969), 206–7.

3. Sweden outlawed burial in churches in 1783. Lindahl, *Grav och rum,* 200.

4. For an examination of the history of bacteriology in Sweden, see Ulrika Graninger, *Från osynligt till synligt: Bakteriologins etablering i sekelskiftets svenska medicin* Stockholm: Carlssons, 1997).

5. The Swedish Cremation Society published its own journal from 1883 onward, under the name *Meddelanden från Svenska Likbrännings-Föreningen*. In 1918 the name was changed to *Meddelanden från Svenska Eldbegängelseföreningen*, and from 1929 onward it was called *Årsmeddelanden från Svenska Eldbegängelseföreningen*. Hereafter, I refer to these publications by the simplified title *Meddelanden*. The journal was published at various intervals until 1929, when it became an annual publication. From the beginning, it contained articles; reports on discussions of cremation in the Swedish Riksdag, at church conferences, in the press, and similar discussions; and information on the society's activities. In the 1920s and especially after 1929, information about the society itself dominated the journal. In 1929 the society also began publishing the magazine *Ignis,* which had a more cultural focus, under the direction of the society's leader, schoolmaster Oscar Övden of Uppsala. Cremation advocates also actively debated in the press, and they published small works essentially written in the genre of popular science, for example, Per Lindell's *Likbränning eller begrafning?*, published as number 32 in the series *Studentföreningen Verdandis småskrifter* (Stockholm, 1891). This chapter of my study is based on an analysis of all editions of *Meddelanden* and *Ignis* up to 1945, as well as other available cremationist literature. From this considerable body of material, I have selected interesting examples to illustrate the arguments used by the movement. Portions of this chapter have been previously published in Åhrén, *Renande lågor.*

6. Curt Wallis, "Om likförbränning," *Hygiea* 4 (1877): 193.

7. Ibid., 198.

8. Richard Wawrinsky, "Huru skola vi lämpligast oskadliggöra menniskolik," *Meddelanden* 4 (1884): 20. See also Ernst Almquist, *Allmän hälsovårdslära: Med särskildt avseende på svenska förhållanden: För läkare, medicine studerande, hälsovårdsmyndigheter, tekniker m. fl.* (Stockholm, 1897). While Almquist, a professor of hygiene at the Karolinska Institute, does indeed report on problems involving earth burial, he is critical of claims that poisons and contagion spread from cemeteries. He felt the hygienic basis for the introduction of cremation in Sweden was immaterial. However, he believed cremation could save space in major cities (chapter 4: "Om liks behandling," 250–61).

9. See Graninger, *Från osynligt till synligt*.

10. F. Levison, "Begrafningsplatserna ur sanitär synpunkt," *Meddelanden* 27 (1900): 23–35.

11. For studies of the history of ideas regarding the role of science in culture and society in turn-of-the-twentieth-century Sweden, see Jonsson, *Vid vetandets gräns; Vetenskapsbärarna,* ed. Sven Widmalm; Eriksson, *Kartläggarna;* Martin Kylhammar, *Maskin och idyll: Teknik och pastorala ideal hos Strindberg och Heidenstam* (Malmö: Liber, 1990).

12. Karin Johannisson, *Medicinens öga: Sjukdom, medicin och samhälle—historiska erfarenheter* (Stockholm: Norstedts, 1990), 64.

13. Eriksson, *Kartläggarna,* 176–78.

14. Jonas Frykman, "På väg—bilder av kultur och klass," in *Modärna tider: Vision och vardag i folkhemmet* eds. Jonas Frykman and Orvar Löfgren (Malmö: Liber, 1985), 74–75.

15. The early evolution of cremation in various countries is studied in detail in Lindell, *Likbränningen jemte öfriga grafskick. Meddelanden* reported annually on the progress of the cremationist cause worldwide. For a comprehensive, comparative, international book on cremation and its many histories, see the *Encyclopedia of Cremation,* ed. Douglas J. Davies, with Lewis H. Mates (Aldershot: Ashgate, 2006). On cremation in Britain and America, see Brian Parsons, *Committed to the Flame: The Development of Cremation in Nineteenth-Century England* (Reading: Spire Books, 2005); Fred Rosen, *Cremation in America* (Amherst, MA: Prometheus Books, 2004); Peter C. Jupp, *From Dust to Ashes: Cremation and the British Way of Death* (Basingstoke: Palgrave Macmillan, 2006); Maria Koskinen; *Burning the Body: The Debate on Cremation in Britain, 1874–1902* (Tampere, Finland: Tampereen Yliopistopaino, 2000); Stephen Prothero, *Purified by Fire: A History of Cremation in America* (Berkeley: University of California Press, 2001).

16. The first municipal crematorium in Sweden was the Sandsborg Crematorium in southern Stockholm, which began operations in 1931 (Enström, *Kyrkan och eldbegängelserörelsen,* 225).

17. For example, see the article signed by E., "Hvad förstås med Likbränning i våra dagar?" *Meddelanden* 1 (1883): 17–19.

18. The lines from Maeterlinck cited here are from *Meddelanden* 65 (1928): 176, in which they were used at the conclusion of an article translated from English, "Folkhälsan och eldbegängelse," by Dr. Allen Daley of Hull.

19. Article by the engineer E. A. Wiman, "Kvinnans förhållande till likbränningsreformen," *Meddelanden* 24 (1897): 35. The article was originally presented as a lecture, but 5,000 copies were also published as a free brochure given to visitors at

the 1897 Scandinavian Exposition of Arts and Industry, where the society had a small display (*Meddelanden* 25 [1898]: 10).

20. Ingeborg Olsson, "Dödens majestät," *Meddelanden* 64 (1927): 141.

21. Ibid.

22. Ibid., 142.

23. Ibid., 144.

24. *Meddelanden* 60 (1923): 26. Regarding Heidenstam as a figurehead for the cremation movement, see Enström, *Kyrkan och eldbegängelserörelsen*, 192–94.

25. *Meddelanden* 65 (1928). The poem was part of Heidenstam's collection of poetry titled *Nya dikter* (1915). It was also published in a facsimile of Heidenstam's handwriting in *Meddelanden* 58 (1923).

26. *Meddelanden* 65 (1928): 177.

27. This poem was written by Peter Rosegger and was given a Swedish interpretation by Kåre Johansson. *Meddelanden* 64 (1927): 145. For a study of death motifs in literature, see Carl Fehrman, *Liemannen, Thanatos och Dödens ängel: Studier i 1700- och 1800-talens litterära ikonologi* (Lund: Gleerup, 1957).

28. For more on cremationist poetry, see Enström, *Kyrkan och eldbegängelserörelsen*, chapter 10.

29. Övden, 275.

30. According to Övden, the Swedish verb *eldbegå* was invented by Hjalmar Samzelius. Ibid., 276.

31. Ibid.

32. The term *krematorium* came into general use in Sweden in the 1930s.

33. Ulf G. Johnsson, "De första svenska krematorierna och deras förutsättningar," *Konsthistorisk tidskrift* 3–4 (1964): 117. See also Emilie Karlsmo, "Rum för begravning: 1900-talets begravningskapell och krematorier," *Tro och tanke* 6 (1998); Karlsmo, *Rum för avsked: Begravningskapellets arkitektur och konstnärliga utsmyckning i 1900-talets Sverige* (Göteborg: Makadam, 2005).

34. The statue was created by Ragnhild Schlyter, Gustav Schlyter's wife, who was a sculptor and created many of the decorative details in the crematorium, which was constructed in 1929. *Meddelanden* 67 (1930).

35. Johnsson, "De första svenska krematorierna,"117.

36. Both Enström and Johnsson also discussed the aesthetic and religious agendas of Schlyter and the Baltic Temple. The term "Romantic" is used to describe an emotional-Romantic religious stance. See Enström, *Kyrkan och eldbegängelserörelsen*, section 2, chapter 1.

37. Within the cremation movement, ideological disagreement existed. Certain members were clearly anti-church, while others sought ties with the church and wanted to tone down the Romantic tendencies sometimes expressed by Gustav Schlyter and others. For a discussion of these issues, see Enström, *Kyrkan och eldbegängelserörelsen*.

38. Ibid.; see the illustration on 401, as well as the discussion regarding the spreading of ashes, 364–67.

39. Ulf G. Johnsson considered this action an odd contradiction of the concept of the purity of cremation and the antipathy its advocates held regarding earth burial (Johnsson, "De första svenska krematorierna," 110). For international comparisons, see *Encyclopedia of Cremation*.

40. Among others, see Oscar Övden, "Skall kistan sänkas vid eldbegängelse?" *Ignis* 2 (1939). Enström takes up this issue in *Kyrkan och eldbegängelserörelsen*, 353–61, and Karlsmo, "Rum för begravning," on 60.

41. However, this practice did not become dominant until the 1970s, according to Karlsmo ("Rum för begravning," 82).

42. Jean-Claude Pressac, *Krematoriene i Auschwitz: Massedrapets maskineri* (Oslo: Aventura, 1994). Thanks to Mats Fridlund for this reference.

43. Cf. Karlsmo, *Rum för begravning*.

44. For international cremation statistics, see *Encyclopedia of Cremation*, 454–56.

45. This matter deserves further study. Roger Cooter also touches briefly on this issue in "The Dead Body," in *Medicine in the Twentieth Century*, ed. Roger Cooter and John Pickstone (Amsterdam: Harwood Academic Publishers, 2000), 474.

46. Gustav Schlyter, "Eldbegängelsens teknik: Det moderna förbränningssystemet," *Meddelanden* 62 (1925): 46.

47. Lindell, *Likbränningen*, 265; Prothero, *Purified by Fire*, chapter 2.

48. Schlyter, "Eldbegängelsens teknik," 50. Schlyter, in turn, took this quotation from a text in which the Höganäs Corporation presented its new furnace, called System Höganäs (the Höganäs System).

49. Henrik Björck, "Bilder av maskiner och ingenjörskårens bildande: Tekniska tidskrifter och introduktion av ny teknik i Sverige, 1800–1870," *Polhem* 5 (1987): esp. 292–93.

50. Ibid., 295–300.

51. Cf. Runeby, *Teknikerna, vetenskapen, och kulturen*, chapter 1.

52. E., "Hvad förstås med likbränning i våra dagar," 18–19. The "E." may stand for Erik Klingenstierna, a military colonel who constructed the first Swedish crematorium incinerator.

53. These two examples are not the only ones; the Cremation Society's publications contain numerous similar statements.

54. *TABO Cremator* (Järfälla, Sweden: Tabo Processionsteknik KB, n.d.), 1. This brochure was included as an addendum to a thesis, "Eldbegängelsens teknikhistoria," by Peter Thomasson, student at the Royal Institute of Technology (KTH), Department for the History of Technology, Stockholm, 1987. Thanks to Professor Svante Lindqvist for this reference.

55. Compare the parallel process that occurred when flush toilets replaced privies: an unhygienic and offensive-smelling device was replaced by a clean, odor-free technology. A technological device offered a solution to a bodily, foul-smelling, and unavoidable phenomenon that had become an urgent sanitary problem, especially in cities.

56. Among others, see Schlyter, "Eldbegängelsens teknik," 54–55; *TABO Cremator*, 1. Schlyter claimed that the crematorium architects of the 1880s "wanted to proudly show off the technology," which he felt was the wrong course of action. The attitude toward technology had clearly changed: in the 1920s technology was still important, but it was not supposed to be prominent. See also Johnsson, 118, 124.

57. This technology was developed by biologist Susanne Wiigh-Mäsak. In the city of Jönköping, the office in charge of cemetery administration has decided to conduct experiments using the new method.

58. KU 2302.

59. Jan-Åke Karlsson, *Eldbegängelse—minneslund, ett kristet begravningssätt?* (Liatorp, 1989).

60. For example, *Meddelanden* 67 (1930): 67.

61. Klintberg, *Råttan i pizzan*, 167–68. This legend seems to have been told from at least the 1930s through the 1970s. Considering that it has to do with Swedish emigration to the United States, it could possibly be even older.

62. Venetia Newall, "Folklore and Cremation," *Folklore* 96, no. 1 (1985). In reality, it is impossible to see any flames from the chapel. First, the casket is not conveyed directly into the incinerator but instead rolls out into another room. Second, in the portion of the incinerator into which the casket is inserted, there is no flame until the incinerator has been closed up—there simply are no flames to see.

63. Ibid., 150–51.

64. See, for example, Schlyter's *Die Halle des Lebens: Die Geschichte eines dreissigjährigen Kampfes für die Umwandlung unserer Friedhöfe und Krematorien in eine Friedensinstitution der Gesellschaft* (Hälsingborg, Sweden, 1938). Here, at the late date of 1938, Schlyter laments that the word *rasse* had fallen out of use in the Baltic Temple agenda. Schlyter's papers, which are preserved at the Lunds Landsarkiv in Lund, include diaries, notebooks, correspondence, and similar documents, all of which deal with cremation. See also Enström, *Kyrkan och eldbegängelserörelsen*, 306.

65. *Meddelanden* 77 (1941): 82, probably translated from German into Swedish by Övden. In 1945, *Ignis* was still publishing texts by Zeiss, and during the war Övden had several articles published in Germany.

66. Information about the society's members is from *Meddelanden*. For this study, all membership lists from 1883 to 1939 were reviewed.

67. For more information on Ada Nilsson and her female medical colleagues, see Nilsson, "Kön, klass, och vetenskaplig auktoritet"; Nilsson, *Kampen om Kvinnan*.

68. "The cremation movement" is an established term, although its relevance is debatable. It was an association with a small core of active initiative-takers and many passive members, as opposed to other folk movements of that era (such as the temperance movement and the labor movement), which were based on broad, active involvement both within and outside the activities of the particular association. However, we can probably refer to the cremation movement of the interwar years as a true folk movement. During this period, the society experienced an increase in both membership and the number of local chapters, established a new insurance plan for members, and gained increased social and cultural openness toward its agenda. For an examination of both conceptual and concrete implications of "movements," see Thörn, *Modernitet, sociologi och sociala rörelser;* Thörn, *Rörelser i det moderna: Politik, modernitet och kollektiv identitet i Europa 1789–1989* (Stockholm: Tiden/Athena, 1997).

69. Karlsmo, "Rum för begravning," 60–62; Enström, *Kyrkan och eldbegängelserörelsen*, 226–27.

70. The British cremation movement felt the same sort of terror regarding the decay of the body. See Jennifer Leaney, "Ashes to Ashes: Cremation and the Celebration of Death in Nineteenth-Century Britain," in *Death, Ritual and Bereavement*, ed. Ralph Houlbrooke (London: Routledge, 1989). Leaney also shows that the themes I have observed in the arguments presented by Swedish cremation advocates were also prevalent in Great Britain, for example, progress, science, purity, beauty, and poetry.

In addition, the British movement had the same radical tendencies, which were sensationalized by the opposition.

71. Karlsmo, "Rum för begravning," 50. For statistics on cremation in Sweden, see *Kyrkogården* 3 (1997); for international statistics, see *Encyclopedia of Cremation*, 456. (The Czech Republic topped the list of Western countries in 2002 with a cremation rate of 77.05 percent, followed by Switzerland at 75.15 percent, Denmark at 72.36 percent, the United Kingdom at 71.89 percent, and Sweden at 70.00 percent. In the United States 27.78 percent of the dead were cremated the same year.)

Chapter Seven

1.   Cf. Young, *Presence in the Flesh*, 127; Metcalf and Huntington, *Celebrations of Death*, introduction; Laderman, *Sacred Remains*, 1.

2.   Julia Kristeva, *Powers of Horror: An Essay on Abjection* (New York: Columbia University Press, 1982 [1980]), 3–4.

3.   Ibid., 2–4.

4.   Cf. Metcalf and Huntington, *Celebrations of Death;* Laderman, *Rest in Peace*, 15–17.

5.   Cf. Walter, *Revival of Death*, chapter 1; David E. Stannard, *The Puritan Way of Death: A Study in Religion, Culture, and Social Change* (Oxford: Oxford University Press, 1977), conclusion.

6.   *Dagens Nyheter* (February 22, 2002). Regarding the development of press photography's relationship with death, see Birna Marianne Kleivan, "Att dø i pressen," *Siden Saxo: Magasin for dansk historie* 4 (1995).

7.   Jonas Frykman, "Clean and Proper: Body and Soul through Peasant and Bourgeois Eyes," in *Culture Builders: A Historical Anthropology of Middle Class Life*, ed. Jonas Frykman and Orvar Löfgren (New Brunswick, NJ: Rutgers University Press, 1987 [1979]), 174.

8.   *Culture Builders*, ed. Frykman and Löfgren, chapter 5, "Peasant Views of Purity and Dirt," especially 174–76.

9.   See Åkesson, *Mellan levande och döda*.

Bibliography

Archives and Collections

Medical Museion, University of Copenhagen
    Iconographical Collection
National Library of Sweden, Stockholm
    Ephemera Collection
    Poster Collection
Nationalmuseum [National Museum of Fine Arts], Stockholm
    Collection of Drawings
    Photo Archive
Nordiska Museet [Nordic Museum], Stockholm
    Folklore Archive
    Etnologiska undersökningen (EU)
    Kulturhistoriska undersökningen (KU)
    N. E. Hammarstedt Archive
    Photographic Collection
Regional State Archives, Lund
    Gustav Schlyter Collection
Royal Swedish Academy of Arts, Stockholm
    Art Collection
Stockholm City Museum
    Photographic Collection
Uppsala University Library
    Maps and Prints

Primary Sources

Interviews

Interview with Sten Didrik Bellander by Anna Tellgren, April 2, 1993. In the possession of Tellgren.
Telephone interviews with professional photographers in Stockholm by the author, February 5, 2000. In the possession of the author.

192   BIBLIOGRAPHY

Published works

Almquist, Ernst. *Allmän hälsovårdslära: Med särskildt avseende på svenska förhållanden: För läkare, medicine studerande, hälsovårdsmyndigheter, tekniker m. fl.* Stockholm: Norstedt, 1897.

———. "Hygieniska institutionen," in *Karolinska mediko-kirurgiska institutets historia,* vol. 3. Stockholm: Isaac Marcus Boktryckeri, 1910.

Årsmeddelanden från Svenska Eldbegängelseföreningen. 1929–39.

Bendz, Hans. "Bidrag till kännedomen om hängningsdödens fenomen," *Lunds universitets årsskrift* 21. Lund, 1885.

Bergstrand, Hilding. *Till frågan om vad som bör innefattas i begreppet mänskligt liv i rättslig mening.* Stockholm: Karolinska institutet, 1916.

Borelius, Jacques. "Om aseptiska operationers utförande i sterila bomullsvantar samt septiska operationers och obduktioners utförande i gummihandskar." *Hygiea* 2 (1898).

Broman, Ivar. *Människohjärnan: En kortfattad handledning vid dess studium och dissektion.* Lund: Gleerup, 1926.

———. *Normale und abnorme Entwicklung des Menshen: Ein Hand- und Lehrbuch der Ontogenie und Teratologie, speziell für praktische Ärzte und Studierende der Medizin.* Wiesbaden, 1911.

———. *Vidunder och missfoster i fantasi och verklighet.* Stockholm: Bonnier, 1929.

Castans anatomiska museum: Katalog öfver Naturvetenskaplig-Anatomiska Afdelningen och Panoptikon-afdelningen. Örebro, Sweden, 1909.

Clason, Edvard. "Huru bör man dissekera? Föreläsning vid öppnandet af den nya dissektionssalen d. 10 Nov. 1884," in *Ordningsreglor för arbetet vid anatomiska institutionen.* Uppsala: Anatomiska institutionen, Uppsala Universitet, 1885.

Daley, Allen. "Folkhälsan och eldbegängelse." *Meddelanden från Svenska Eldbegängelseföreningen* 65 (1928).

E. "Hvad förstås med Likbränning i våra dagar?" *Meddelanden från Svenska Eldbegängelseföreningen* 1 (1883).

Författningar m.m. angående medicinalväsendet i Sverige omfattande tiden från och med 1860 till och med år 1876, förra delen (1860–1873), ed. A Kullberg. Stockholm 1877.

Författningar m.m. angående medicinalväsendet i Sverige omfattande tiden från och med år 1877 till och med år 1882, ed. D. M. Pontin. Stockholm, 1884.

Författningar m.m. angående medicinalväsendet i Sverige omfattande år 1886, ed. D. M. Pontin. Stockholm, 1887.

Författningar m.m. angående medicinalväsendet i Sverige omfattande år 1888, ed. D. M. Pontin. Stockholm, 1889.

Förhandlingar vid Svenska Läkaresällskapets Sammankomster. Stockholm, 1870–1901.

Fürst, Carl M. "Professorn i Fysiologi vid Lunds universitet Magnus Blix' hjärna," in *Lunds universitets årsskrift,* part 2, vol. 14, no. 3. Lund, 1918.

Gadelius, Bror. "Om förhållandet mellan psykiatri och hjärnanatomi: Installationsföreläsning hållen vid Karolinska Institutet den 16 mars 1904," in *Allmänna Svenska Läkartidningen.* Stockholm, 1904.

Handlingar rörande Norbergska målet, del I: Rättegångshandlingar från rådhusrätten i Gefle. Lund: Gleerup, 1897.

Heidenstam, Verner von. "Bön vid lågorna." *Meddelanden från Svenska Eldbegängelse-föreningen* 65 (1928).

Henschen, Salomon Eberhard. "Om den tekniska undersökningen af hjärnan: Några anmärkningar," in *Festskrift tillegnad direktören och öfverläkaren vid Sabbatsbergs sjukhus med doktorn F. W. Warfvinge vid fylda 60 år.* Stockholm: Samson & Wallin, 1894.

Hofmann, Eduard Ritter von. *Atlas der gerichtlichen Medizin.* München: Lehmann, 1889.

———. *Rättsmedicinsk atlas.* Stockholm: Bille, 1898 [1889].

Holmgren, Emil. *Lärobok i histologi.* Stockholm: Norstedt, 1920.

Holmgren, Frithiof. "Om halshuggning betraktad från fysiologisk synpunkt," in *Uppsala Läkaresällskaps förhandlingar,* vol. 2, 1875–76. Uppsala, 1876.

Holmgren, Israel. *Mitt liv,* vols. 1–2. Stockholm: Natur och kultur, 1959.

Huss, Magnus. *Några skizzer och tidsbilder från min lefnad: Hämtade dels från äldre anteckningar, dels ur minnet vid 78 års ålder.* Stockholm: Norstedt, 1891.

Hvar 8:e dag. 1899–1932.

Hygiea: Medicinsk och farmaceutisk månadsskrift. 1870–1938.

Ignis, tidskrift för eldbegängelsespörsmål. 1929–38.

Karlsson, Jan-Åke. *Eldbegängelse—minneslund, ett kristet begravningssätt?* Liatorp, Sweden, 1989.

Karolinska mediko-kirurgiska institutets historia, vols. 1–3. Stockholm: Isaac Marcus Boktryckeri, 1910.

Katalog N:o I öfver patologiska afdelningen och Naturfenomenen [N. Nielséns Panoptikon]. Stockholm, 1863.

Katalog öfver Det stora Etnologiska, Geologiska, Anatomiska, Fysiologiska, Embryologiska och Patologiska Museum. Stockholm, 1863.

Katalog öfver Linu's internationella panoptikon och anatomiska vaxmuseum. Örebro, Sweden, 1914.

Key, Axel. *Till kirurgins historia i Sverige.* Stockholm, 1897.

Key-Åberg, Algot. *För obduktionsbordet: Författningar och protokoll jämte utlåtanden.* Stockholm: Norstedt, 1916.

———. "Gällande bestämmelser rörande tillgången till lik för den anatomiska undervisningen i Stockholm, Uppsala och Lund." *Hygiea* (1889).

———. "Rätts- och statsmedicinska institutionen," in *Karolinska mediko-kirurgiska institutets historia,* vol. 3. Stockholm: Isaac Marcus Boktryckeri, 1910.

Levison, F. "Begrafningsplatserna ur sanitär synpunkt." *Meddelanden från Svenska Likbränningsföreningen* 27 (1900).

Lindell, Per. *Likbränning eller begrafning?* Stockholm: Bonnier, 1891.

———. *Likbränningen jemte öfriga grafskick.* Stockholm, 1888.

Lovén, Christian. "Om lymfvägar i magsäckens slemhinna," in *Nordiskt medicinskt arkiv,* vol. 5, no. 26. Stockholm, 1873.

Meddelanden från Svenska Eldbegängelseföreningen. 1918–28.

Meddelanden från Svenska Likbränningsföreningen. 1883–1917.

Müller, Erik. "Anatomiska institutionen," in *Karolinska mediko-kirurgiska institutets historia,* vol. 3. Stockholm: Isaac Marcus Boktryckeri, 1910.

———. "Några ord om anatomien såsom vetenskap och läroämne." *Hygiea* 2 (1899).

Norberg, Johan Petrus. *Medicinska rättsfallet i Gefle 1896*. Gävle, Sweden: Ekmans förlagsexped., 1897.

Ny illustrerad tidning: För konst, bildning och nöje. 1880–1900.

Öhrvall, Hjalmar. *Den fysiologiska döden och dess betydelse för lifvet*. Stockholm: Skoglund, 1899.

Olsson, Ingeborg. "Dödens majestät." *Meddelanden från Svenska Eldbegängelseföreningen* 64 (1927).

Övden, Oscar. *Eldbegängelsen—framtidens gravskick*. Stockholm: Seelig, 1929.

———. *Eldbegängelsens historia i Sverige 1882–1932*. Stockholm: Svenska Eldbegängelseföreningen, 1932.

———. "Skall kistan sänkas vid eldbegängelse?" *Ignis* 2 (1939).

Petrén, Viktor. "Reformerad begravningsverksamhet i Stockholm." *Ignis* 1 (1946).

Quensel, Ulrik. "Om en ny metod att konservera anatomiska preparat med bibehållandet af de naturliga färgerna." *Hygiea* 9 (1897).

———. "Ytterligare några ord om en ny metod att konservera anatomiska preparat med bibehållandet af de naturliga färgerna." *Hygiea* 11 (1897).

Reclam, Carl. *Menniskokroppen, dess byggnad och lif: Populära föredrag*. Stockholm: Ad. Bonnier, 1884.

Retzius, Gustaf. *Biologische Untersuchungen, Neue Folge*, vols. 1–19. Stockholm, Leipzig, Jena, 1890–1921.

———. "Om metoderna att konservera hjärnor," in *Biologiska föreningens förhandlingar*, vol. 1, no. 6. Stockholm, 1889.

———. "Joseph Hyrtl." *Hygiea* 2 (1894).

———. *Das Menschenhirn: Studien in der makroskopische Morphologie*. Stockholm, 1896.

———. *Biografiska anteckningar och minnen*, ed. O. Walde, vol. 1–2. Uppsala: 1933–48.

Samling av författningar och cirkulär m.m. angående medicinalväsendet, serie A. Stockholm: Kungl. Medicinalstyrelsen, 1926 and 1932.

Schlyter, Gustav. "Eldbegängelsens teknik: Det moderna förbränningssystemet." *Meddelanden från Svenska Eldbegängelseföreningen* 62 (1925).

———. *Die Feuerbestattung und ihre kulturelle Bedeutung: Der Tempel des Friedens*. Leipzig: Wilh. Hemp, 1922.

———. *Die Halle des Lebens: Die Geschichte eines dreissigjährigen Kampfes für die Umwandlung unserer Friedhöfe und Krematorien in eine Friedensinstitution der Gesellschaft*. Hälsingborg, Sweden: Hälsingborgs litogr.,1938.

Sjövall, Einar. *Om döden, en biologisk överblick*. Lund: Gleerup, 1915.

Sundberg, Carl. "Patologisk-anatomiska institutionen," in *Karolinska mediko-kirurgiska institutets historia*, vol. 3. Stockholm: Isaac Marcus Boktryckeri, 1922.

Svenska Panoptikons Vägvisare. Stockholm, 1922.

Sveriges Begravningsentreprenörers Förbund. *Års-och Revisionsberättelse för år 1931: Protokoll över årsmötet den 17 juli 1932*. [Stockholm]: 1932.

TABO Cremator. Järfälla, Sweden: Tabo Procesionsteknik KB, n.d.

Uppsala universitet: Anatomiska institutionen: Ordningsreglor för arbetet vid den anatomiska instutionen 1885. Uppsala: Uppsala universitet, 1885.

Vägvisare genom Svenska Panoptikon. Stockholm, 1894, 1895, 1922.

Wallis, Curt. "Om likförbränning." *Hygiea* 4 (1877).

Wawrinsky, Richard. "Huru skola vi lämpligast oskadliggöra menniskolik?" *Meddelanden från Svenska Likbränningsföreningen* 24 (1897).

Wilén, Brynhild. *Folkminnessamlingen: Död och begravning,* vol. 1. Nordic Museum Archives (NMA), recorded in 1928.

Wiman, E. A. "Kvinnans förhållande till likbränningsreformen." *Meddelanden från Svenska Likbränningsföreningen* 24 (1897).

Secondary Sources

Adams, Sheila. "A Gendered History of the Social Management of Death in Foleshill, Coventry, during the Interwar Years," in *The Sociology of Death: Theory, Culture, Practice,* ed. David Clark. Oxford: Blackwell, 1993.

Ahlström, Carl Gustaf. "Arvid Florman—den förste patologen i Lund," in *Sydsvenska medicinhistoriska sällskapets årsskrift.* Lund, 1975.

———. "Ett gammalt museum berättar: Glimtar från patologiska institutionens museum i Lund," in *Sydsvenska medicinhistoriska sällskapets årsskrift.* Lund, 1982.

———. "Patologisk anatomi i Lund 1668–1962," in *Sydsvenska medicinhistoriska sällskapets årsskrift,* supplementum 2. Lund, 1983.

Åhrén, Eva. "Aspekter på döden i det moderna samhället." Unpublished master's thesis, Stockholm, Avdelningen för idéhistoria, Stockholms universitet, 1994.

———. *Renande lågor: Den svenska eldbegängelserörelsens framväxt under 1800-talets sista decennier.* Stockholm: Avdelningen för idéhistoria, Stockholms universitet, 1994.

Åhrén Snickare, Eva. *Döden, kroppen och moderniteten.* Stockholm: Carlssons, 2002.

———. "Känn dig själv: Om vaxkabinett och anatomiska utställningar," in *Den mediala vetenskapen,* ed. Anders Ekström. Nora, Sweden: Nya Doxa, 2004.

———. "Kroppar av vax: Modeller och preparat i konst och vetenskap," in *Kroppen: Konst och vetenskap,* ed. Lena Holger. Stockholm: Nationalmuseum, 2005.

———. "Människokroppen som spektakel: Om vaxkabinett och deras marknadsföring kring sekelskiftet 1900," in *Reklam och hälsa: Levnadsideal, skönhet och hälsa i den svenska reklamens historia,* ed. Roger Qvarsell and Ulrika Torell. Stockholm: Carlssons, 2005.

———. "Minnesbilder: Om fotografier av de döda," in *Visuella spår: Bilder i kultur- och samhällsanalys,* ed. Eva Åhrén Snickare, Anna Sparrman, and Ulrika Torell. Lund: Studentlitteratur, 2003.

Åkesson, Lynn. "Döda kroppars budskap," in *Kroppens tid: Om samspelet mellan kropp, identitet och samhälle,* ed. Susanne Lundin and Lynn Åkesson. Stockholm: Natur och kultur, 1996.

———. "Dödens rationalitet och mystik," in *Döden i Ystad.* Ystad, Sweden: Ystads Museer, 1994.

———. *Mellan levande och döda: Föreställningar om kropp och ritual.* Stockholm: Natur och Kultur, 1997.

Åkesson, Lynn, and Susanne Lundin. "Att skapa liv och utforska död." *Kulturella perspektiv* 1 (1995).

Alasuutari, Pertti. *Researching Culture: Qualitative Method and Cultural Studies.* London: Sage, 1995.

The Anatomical Waxes of La Specola, ed. Joseph Renahan. Florence, Italy: Arnaud 1995.

Ander, Karl-Erik O-n. *Helsingborgs första fotografer och deras bilder 1840–1900.* Helsingborg, Sweden: K. E. O-n Ander, 1998.

Andersson, Lars M., Lars Berggren, and Ulf Zander, eds. *Mer än tusen ord: Bilden och de historiska vetenskaperna.* Lund: Historiska Media, 2001.

Ansikte mot ansikte: Porträtt från fem sekel, ed. Görel Cavalli-Björkman. Stockholm: Nationalmuseum/Atlantis, 2001.

Ariès, Philippe. *Essais sur l'histoire de la mort en Occident.* Paris: Éditions du Seuil, 1971.

———. *Homme devant la mort.* Paris: Éditions du Seuil, 1977.

———. *The Hour of Our Death.* Oxford: Oxford University Press, 1991 [1977].

———. *Images de l'homme devant la mort.* Paris: Éditions du Seuil, 1983.

———. *Images of Man and Death.* Cambridge, MA: Harvard University Press, 1985.

———. *Western Attitudes toward Death: From the Middle Ages to the Present.* Baltimore: Johns Hopkins University Press, 1974.

Barthes, Roland. *Camera Lucida: Reflections on Photography.* New York: Hill and Wang, 1981 [1980].

Bauman, Zygmunt. *Mortality, Immortality, and Other Life Strategies.* Cambridge, UK: Polity, 1992.

Becker, Karin. "Picturing Our Past: An Archive Constructs a National Culture." *Journal of American Folklore* 105, no. 415 (1992).

Beckman, Jenny. *Naturens palats: Nybyggnad, vetenskap och utställning vid Naturhistoriska riksmuseet 1866–1925.* Stockholm: Atlantis, 1999.

Bendann, E[ffie]. *Death Customs: An Analytical Study of Burial Rites.* London: Kegan Paul, 1930.

Bennett, Tony. *The Birth of the Museum: History, Theory, Politics.* London: Routledge, 1995.

———. "Pedagogic Objects, Clean Eyes, and Popular Instruction: On Sensory Regimes and Museum Didactics." *Configurations: A Journal of Literature, Science, and Technology* 6, no. 3 (1998).

Berman, Marshall. *All That Is Solid Melts into Air: The Experience of Modernity.* New York: Simon and Schuster, 1982.

Beyond the Cultural Turn: New Directions in the Study of Society and Culture, ed. Victoria E. Bonnell and Lynn Hunt. Berkeley: University of California Press, 1999.

Björck, Henrik. "Bilder av maskiner och ingenjörskårens bildande: Tekniska tidskrifter och introduktion av ny teknik i Sverige, 1800–1870." *Polhem* 5 (1987).

Bocock, Robert. "The Cultural Formations of Modern Society," in *Modernity: An Introduction to Modern Societies,* ed. S. Hall, D. Held, D. Hubert, and K. Thompson. Cambridge, MA: Blackwell, 1996.

The Body: Social Process and Cultural Theory, ed. Mike Featherstone, Mike Hepworth, and Brian Turner. London: Sage, 1992.

Bogdan, Robert. *Freak Show: Presenting Human Oddities for Amusement and Profit.* Chicago: University of Chicago Press, 1988.

Bondeson, Jan. *Medicinhistoriskt kuriosakabinett: Essayer.* Kivik, Sweden: Kiviksgårdens förlag, 1992.

Bonds, Gonvor. *Anatomier: Studieteckningar ur Konstakademiens samlingar.* Stockholm: Kungl. Akademien för de fria konsterna, 1991.

Bremborg, Anna Davidsson. "Från stigmatisering till professionalisering? En studie av begravningsentreprenörer utifrån ett aktörsperspektiv." Master's thesis, Lund, Lund University, 2000.

———. "Vem tar hand om den döda kroppen? Om genusarbetsfördelning på begravningsbyråer," in *Stigma, status och strategier: Genusperspektiv i religionsvetenskap*, ed. Catharina Raudvere. Lund: Studentlitteratur, 2002.

———. *Yrke: begravningsentreprenör: Om utanförskap, döda kroppar, riter och professionalisering*. Lund: Studentlitteratur, 2002.

Brey, Philip. "Theorizing Modernity and Technology," in *Modernity and Technology*, ed. T. J. Misa, P. Brey, and A. Feenberg. Cambridge, MA: MIT Press, 2003.

Bringéus, Nils-Arvid. *Klockringningsseden i Sverige*. Stockholm: Nordiska Museets förlag, 1958.

———. *Livets högtider*. Stockholm: LT, 1987.

———. *Människan som kulturvarelse: En introduktion till etnologin*. Stockholm: Carlssons, 1990 [1976].

———. *Svensk begravningssed i historisk belysning*. Fonus, 1986.

———. "Vår hållning till döden, speglad genom begravninsseden förr och nu," in *Vår hållning till döden*, ed. Erik Bylund. Umeå, Sweden: CEWE-förlaget/Erik Bylund, 1983.

———. "Vår hållning till döden," in *Dödens riter*, ed. Kristina Söderpalm. Stockholm: Carlssons, 1994.

Broberg, Gunnar. "Det antropologiska fotoalbumet," in *Mer än tusen ord: Bilden och de historiska vetenskaperna*, ed. Lars M. Andersson, Lars Berggren, and Ulf Zander. Lund: Nordic Academic Press, 2001.

———. "En kulturanatom: Carl-Herman Hjortsjö," in *Kulturanatomiska studier, Ugglan* no. 15. Lund: Avdelningen för idé- och lärdomshistoria, Lunds universitet, 2001.

———. "Entrébiljett till en skandal." *Tvärsnitt* 1–2 (1991).

———. "Lappkaravaner på villovägar: Antropologin och synen på samerna fram mot sekelskiftet 1900." *Lychnos* (1981–82).

Broberg, Gunnar, and Sverker Sörlin. "Umgänget med muserna." *Tvärsnitt* 1–2 (1991).

Broberg, Gunnar, and Matthias Tydén. *Oönskade i folkhemmet: Rashygien och sterilisering i Sverige*. Stockholm: Gidlunds, 1991.

Broby-Johansens, Rudolf. *Dagens dont i Norden: Arbejdsbilledets historie i Danmark, Norge, Sverige, Finland, Island, på Færøerne, i Grønland og hos samerne*. Aarhus, Denmark: Fremad, 1972.

Bronfen, Elisabeth. *Over Her Dead Body: Death, Femininity, and the Aesthetic*. Manchester: Manchester University Press, 1992.

Burns, Stanley. *Sleeping Beauty: Memorial Photography in America*. New York: Twelvetrees, 1990.

Bynum, W. F. and Roy Porter, eds. *Medicine and the Five Senses*. Cambridge: Cambridge University Press, 1993.

Cartwright, Lisa. *Screening the Body: Tracing Medicine's Visual Culture*. Minneapolis: University of Minnesota Press, 1995.

Christensson, Jacob. "Sven Nilsson och Skandinaviens urinvånare," in *Kulturanatomiska studier, Ugglan* no. 15. Lund: Avdelningen för idé- och lärdomshistoria, Lunds universitet, 2001.

Companion Encyclopedia of the History of Medicine, vols. 1–2, ed. W. F. Bynum and Roy Porter. London: Routledge, 1993.

Cooter, Roger. "The Dead Body," in *Medicine in the Twentieth Century*, ed. Roger Cooter and John Pickstone. Amsterdam: Harwood Academic Publishers, 2000.

Crary, Jonathan. *Suspensions of Perception: Attention, Spectacle, and Modern Culture.* Cambridge, MA: MIT Press, 1999.

———. *Techniques of the Observer: On Vision and Modernity in the Nineteenth Century.* Cambridge, MA: MIT Press, 1999 [1992].

Dagens Nyheter. September 16, 1999; February 22, 2002.

Daston, Lorraine, and Katharine Park. *Wonders and the Order of Nature 1150–1750.* New York: Zone Books, 2001.

Death, Ritual, and Bereavement, ed. Ralph Houlbrooke. London: Routledge, 1989.

Delmas, André. "Le Musée Orfila et le Musée Rouvière." *Surgical and Radiologic Anatomy: Journal of Clinical Anatomy* 17, supplement 1 (1995).

Dijkstra, Bram. *Idols of Perversity: Fantasies of Female Evil in Fin-de-siècle Culture.* New York: Oxford University Press, 1986.

Djurberg, Vilhelm. *När det var anatomisal på Södermalms stadshus i Stockholm 1685–1748.* Stockholm: Norstedts, 1927.

Dödens Riter, ed. Kristina Söderpalm. Stockholm: Carlssons, 1994.

Douglas, Mary. *Purity and Danger: An Analysis of the Concepts of Pollution and Taboo.* London: Routledge, 1996 [1966].

Edström, Per Simon. *Mördaren och helvetesmaskinen: En egensinnig anteckningsbok om en flerårig detektivundersökning av ett resande vaxkabinett och vaxkabinetten i Norden.* Värmdö, Sweden: Arena Theatre Institute, 2005.

———. "Spåren av vaxkabinettet," in *Ett resande vaxkabinett.* Stockholm: Statens historiska museum, 1999.

1897: Mediehistorier kring Stockholmsutställningen, ed. Anders Ekström, Solveig Jülich, and Pelle Snickars. Stockholm: Statens ljud- och bildarkiv, 2006.

Ekenstam, Claes. *Kroppens idéhistoria: Disciplinering och karaktärsdaning i Sverige 1700–1950.* Hedemora, Sweden: Gidlunds, 1993.

Eklöf, Motzi. *Läkarens ethos: Studier i den svenska läkarkårens identiteter, intressen och ideal 1890–1960.* Linköping, Sweden: Institutionen för Tema, Linköpings universitet, 2000.

Ekström, Anders. *Den utställda världen: Stockholmsutställningen 1897 och 1800-talets världsutställningar.* Stockholm: Nordiska museets förlag, 1994.

———. "Förväntningshorisonter, ca. 1870–1920," in *Vetenskapsbärarna: Naturvetenskapen i det svenska samhället, 1880–1950*, ed. Sven Widmalm. Hedemora: Gidlunds, 1999.

———. *Dödens exempel: Självmordstolkningar i svenskt 1800-tal genom berättelsen om Otto Landgren.* Stockholm: Atlantis, 2000.

———. "Konsten att se ett landskapspanorama: Om åskådningspedagogik och exemplarisk realism under 1800-talet," in *Publika kulturer: Att tilltala allmänheten 1700–1900: En inledning.* Uppsala: Institutionen för idé- och lärdomshistoria, Uppsala universitet, 2000.

Encyclopedia of Cremation, ed. Douglas J. Davies, with Lewis H. Mates. Aldershot: Ashgate, 2006.

Enström, Bengt. *Kyrkan och eldbegängelserörelsen i Sverige 1882–1962.* Lund: Gleerup, 1964.

Eriksson, Bengt Erik, and Eva Palmblad. *Kropp och politik: Hälsoupplysning som samhällsspegel från 30-tal till 90-tal.* Stockholm: Carlssons, 1995.

Eriksson, Gunnar. *Kartläggarna: Naturvetenskapens tillväxt och tillämpningar i det industriella genombrottets Sverige 1870–1914.* Umeå, Sweden: Umeå universitet, 1978.

Ett resande vaxkabinett, ed. Inga Lundström and Katarina Svensson. Stockholm: Statens historiska museum, 1999.

Evans, Richard J. *Rituals of Retribution: Capital Punishment in Germany 1600–1987.* Oxford: Oxford University Press, 1996.

Fehrman, Carl. *Kyrkogårdsromantik.* Lund: Gleerup, 1954.

———. *Liemannen, Thanatos och Dödens ängel: Studier i 1700- och 1800-talens litterära ikonologi.* Lund: Gleerup, 1957.

Foucault, Michel. *The Birth of the Clinic: An Archaeology of Medical Perception.* New York: Vintage Books, 1994 [1963].

Freakery: Cultural Spectacles of the Extraordinary Body, ed. Rosemarie Garland Thompson. New York: New York University Press, 1996.

Fredbärj, Telemak. "De offentliga anatomierna i Sverige under 1600- och 1700-talen," in *Medicinhistorisk årsbok 1958.* Stockholm: Medicinhistoriska museet, 1958.

Freedberg, David. *The Power of Images: Studies in the History and Theory of Response.* Chicago: University of Chicago Press, 1989.

French, Roger. "The Anatomical Tradition," in *Companion Encyclopedia of the History of Medicine,* ed. W. F. Bynum and Roy Porter. London: Routledge, 1993.

Frykman, Jonas. "Clean and Proper: Body and Soul through Peasant and Bourgeois Eyes," in *Culture Builders: A Historical Anthropology of Middle Class Life,* ed. Jonas Frykman and Orvar Löfgren. New Brunswick, NJ: Rutgers University Press, 1987 [1979].

———. "På väg—bilder av kultur och klass," in *Modärna tider: Vision och vardag i folkhemmet,* ed. Jonas Frykman and Orvar Löfgren. Malmö, Sweden: Liber, 1985.

The Funeral Effigies of Westminster Abbey, ed. Anthony Harvey and Richard Mortimer. Woodbridge, UK: Boydell, 1994.

Garnert, Jan. *Anden i lampan: Etnologiska perspektiv på ljus och mörker.* Stockholm: Carlssons, 1993.

———. "Rethinking Visual Representation: Notes on the Folklorist and Photographer Nils Keyland." *Nordisk Museologi* 2 (1995).

Gatrell, V.A.C. *The Hanging Tree: Execution and the English People 1770–1868.* Oxford: Oxford University Press, 1994.

Geertz, Clifford. "Thick Description: Toward an Interpretive Theory of Culture," in *The Interpretation of Cultures.* London: Fontana, 1993 [1973].

Gennep, Arnold van. *Les rites de passage: Etude systématique des rites.* Paris: É. Nourry, 1909.

Giddens, Anthony. *The Consequences of Modernity.* Stanford: Stanford University Press, 1990.

Gorer, Geoffrey. "The Pornography of Death." *Encounter* (October 1955).

Graninger, Ulrika. *Från osynligt till synligt: Bakteriologins etablering i sekelskiftets svenska medicin.* Stockholm: Carlssons, 1997.

A Guide to the Hunterian Museum: Bicentenary Edition [Elizabeth Allen]. London: Royal College of Surgeons, 1993.

Gustafsson, Hjördis. "Med karameller och entusiasm som trollmedel: Om folklivsforskaren Louise Hagbergs arbete på 1920-talet." Unpublished thesis, Stockholm, Institutet för folklivsforksning, Stockholms universitet, 1992.

Gustafsson, Tony. *Läkaren, döden och brottet: Studier i den svenska rättsmedicinens etablering.* Uppsala: Acta Universitatis Upsaliensis, 2007.

Gustafsson, Torbjörn. "Frithiof Holmgren och straffanatomin." *Tvärsnitt* 2 (1995).

———. *Själens biologi: Medicinen, kulturen och naturens ordning 1850–1920.* Stockholm: Symposion, 1996.

Habermas, Jürgen. *The Structural Transformation of the Public Sphere.* Cambridge, MA: MIT Press, 1989.

Hafsteinsson, Sigurjón Baldur. "Post-mortem and Funeral Photography in Iceland." *History of Photography* (Spring 1999).

Hagberg, Louise. *När döden gästar: Svenska folkseder och svensk folktro i samband med död och begravning.* Stockholm: Wahlström och Widstrand, 1937.

Hansson, Hertha. *Alkemi, romantik och rasvetenskap: Om en vetenskaplig tradition.* Nora, Sweden: Nya Doxa, 1994.

Hedberg, Gunnel. "Straffet offentligen ske på hans bild och efterliknelse: Några anteckningar till ett lagförslag 1696 om införande av avrättning in effigie i Sverige." *RIG: Kulturhistorisk tidskrift grundad 1918,* 1 (1998).

Henschen, Folke. *Patologings historia i Stockholm.* Stockholm: Almqvist and Wiksell International, 1977.

History of Photography 3, (Spring 1999).

Holme, Lotta. *Konsten att göra barn raka: Ortopedi och vanförevård i Sverige till 1920.* Stockholm: Carlssons, 1996.

Hopwood, Nick. *Embryos in Wax: Models from the Ziegler Studio.* Cambridge: Whipple Museum for the History of Science, University of Cambridge, 2002.

I framtidens tjänst: Ur folkhemmets idéhistoria, ed. Roger Qvarsell. Stockholm: Gidlunds, 1986.

I skuggan av ljuset: Fotografi och systematik i konst, vetenskap och vardagsliv. Stockholm: Moderna museet, 1998.

Inger, Göran. "Rätten över eget liv och över egen kropp," in *Kungl. Humanistiska Vetenskapssamfundet i Uppsala: Årsbok 1985.* Uppsala: Uppsala universitet, 1986.

Jaensson, Gabrielle, and Inga Kindblom. *Kring livets högtider i Örkelljunga församling.* Lund: Gleerup, 1968.

Jameson, Fredric. *A Singular Modernity: Essay on the Ontology of the Present.* London: Verso, 2002.

Jarrick, Arne. *Hamlets fråga: En svensk självmordshistoria.* Stockholm: Norstedts, 2000.

Jensen, Johanne Maria. *Gennem lys og skygger: Familiefotografier fra forrige århundrede til idag.* Herning, Denmark: Systime, 1994.

———. "Livet og døden i familiealbumet." *Siden Saxo: Magasin for dansk historie* 4 (1995).

Johannesson, Lena. *Den massproducerade bilden: Ur bildindustrialismens historia.* Stockholm: Carlssons, 1997 [1978].

————. "Pictures as News, News as Pictures: A Survey of Mass-Reproduced Images in 19ᵗʰ Century Sweden," in *Visual Paraphrases: Studies in Mass Media Imagery*. Uppsala: Uppsala Universitet, 1984.

————. *Mörkrum och transparens: Studier i europeisk bildkultur och i bildens historiska evidens*. Stockholm: Carlssons, 2001.

Johannisson, Karin. *Den mörka kontinenten: Kvinnan, medicinen och fin-de-siècle*. Stockholm: Norstedts, 1994.

————. *Kroppens tunna skal: Sex essäer om kropp, historia och kultur*. Stockholm: Norstedts, 1997.

————. *Medicinens öga: Sjukdom, medicin och samhälle—historiska erfarenheter*. Stockholm: Norstedts, 1990.

Johnsson, Ulf G. "De första svenska krematorierna och deras förutsättningar." *Konsthistorisk tidskrift* 3–4 (1964).

Jonsson, Kjell. "En nybadad renrasig svensk . . . ," in *I framtidens tjänst: ur folkhemmets idéhistoria*, ed. Roger Qvarsell. Stockholm: Gidlunds, 1986.

————. *Harmoni eller konflikt? En idéhistorisk introduktion till förhållandet mellan vetenskap och religion i Västerlandet*. Stockholm: Carlssons, 1991.

————. *Vid vetandets gräns: Om skiljelinjen mellan naturvetenskap och metafysik i svensk kulturdebatt 1870–1920*. Lund: Arkiv, 1987.

Jordanova, Ludmilla. "Medicine and Visual Culture." *The Social History of Medicine* 3 (1990).

————. "Museums: Representing the Real?" in *Realism and Representation: Essays on the Problem of Realism in Relation to Science, Literature, and Culture*, ed. George Levine. Madison: University of Wisconsin Press, 1993.

————. "Objects of Knowledge: A Historical Perspective on Museums," in *The New Museology*, ed. Peter Vergo. London: Reaktion Books, 1989.

————. *Sexual Visions: Images of Gender in Science and Medicine between the Eighteenth and Twentieth Centuries*. Madison: University of Wisconsin Press, 1989.

Jülich, Solveig. "Medicinen och fotografiets mekaniska objektivitet: Carl Curman och tillkomsten av Karolinska institutets fotografiska ateljé 1861," in *Lychnos: Årsbok för idé- och lärdomshistoria*. Uppsala, 1998.

————. *Skuggor av sanning: Tidig svensk radiologi och visuell kultur*. Linköping, Sweden: Institutionen för Tema, Linköpings universitet, 2002.

Jupp, Peter C. *From Dust to Ashes: Cremation and the British Way of Death*. Basingstoke: Palgrave Macmillan, 2006.

Kaiserfeld Thomas, ed. *Från moderna helgonkulter till självmord: Föredrag från Idé- och vetenskapshistorisk konferens 1995*. Stockholm: Avdelningen för teknik-och vetenskapshistoria, KTH, 1995.

Karlsmo, Emilie. *Rum för avsked: Begravningskapellets arkitektur och konstnärliga utsmyckning i 1900-talets Sverige*. Göteborg: Makadam, 2005.

————. "Rum för begravning: 1900-talets begravningskapell och krematorier." *Tro och tanke* 6 (1998).

Karlsson, Eva-Lena. KAT. NR. 313, *Ansikte mot ansikte: Porträtt från fem sekel*, ed. Görel Cavalli Björkman. Stockholm: Nationalmuseum/Atlantis, 2001.

Karolinska mediko-kirurgiska institutets historia, vols. 1–3. Stockholm: Isaac Marcus Boktryckeri, 1910.

Kemp, Martin. "'The Mark of Truth': Looking and Learning in Some Anatomical Illustrations from the Renaissance and Eighteenth Century," in *Medicine and the Five Senses*, ed. W. F. Bynum and Roy Porter. Cambridge: Cambridge University Press, 1993.

———. "Medicine in View: Art and Visual Representation," in *Western Medicine: An Illustrated History*, ed. Irvine Loudon. Oxford: Oxford University Press, 1997.

———. "Temples of the Body and Temples of the Cosmos: Vision and Visualization in the Vesalian and Copernican Revolutions," in *Picturing Knowledge: Historical and Philosophical Problems Concerning the Use of Art in Science*, ed. Brian S. Baigrie. Toronto: University of Toronto Press, 1996.

Kemp, Martin, and Marina Wallace. *Spectacular Bodies: The Art and Science of the Human Body from Leonardo to Now*. Berkeley and London: University of California Press and Hayward Gallery, 2000.

Kern, Stephen. *The Culture of Time and Space, 1880–1918*. Cambridge, MA: Harvard University Press, 2003 [1983].

Kildegaard, Bjarne. "Unlimited Memory: Photography and the Differentiation of Familiar Intimacy," in *Man and Picture: Papers from the First International Symposium for Ethnological Picture Research in Lund 1984*, ed. Nils-Arvid Bringéus. Stockholm: Almqvist and Wiksell International, 1986.

Kleivan, Birna Marianne. "Att dø i pressen." *Siden Saxo: Magasin for dansk historie* 4 (1995).

Klintberg, Bengt af. *Råttan i pizzan: Folksägner i vår tid*. Stockholm: Norstedts, 1986.

Koskinen, Maria. *Burning the Body: The Debate on Cremation in Britain, 1874–1902*. Tampere, Finland: Tampereen Yliopistopaino, 2000.

Kristensson, Hjördis. *Vetenskapens byggnader under 1800-talet: Lund och Europa*. Stockholm: Arkitekturmuseum, 1990.

Kristeva, Julia. *Powers of Horror: An Essay on Abjection*. New York: Columbia University Press, 1982 [1980].

Kroppen efter döden: Slutbetänkande av transplantationsutredningen. SOU (Statens offentliga utredningar) 16. Stockholm: Allmänna förlaget, 1992.

Kübler-Ross, Elisabeth. *On Death and Dying*. New York: Macmillan, 1969.

Kulturanatomiska studier, Ugglan 15. Lund: Avdelningen för idé- och lärdomshistoria, Lunds universitet, 2001.

Kylhammar, Martin. *Maskin och idyll: Teknik och pastorala ideal hos Strindberg och Heidenstam*. Malmö, Sweden: Liber, 1985.

Laderman, Gary. *Rest in Peace: A Cultural History of Death and the Funeral Home in Twentieth Century America*. Oxford: Oxford University Press, 2003.

———. *The Sacred Remains: American Attitudes toward Death, 1799–1883*. New Haven: Yale University Press, 1996.

Lagerkvist, Ulf. *Karolinska institutet och kampen mot universiteten*. Hedemora, Sweden: Gidlunds, 1999.

Lahtinen, Tuomo. *Kremering i Finland: Idéhistoria och utveckling*. Åbo, Finland: Åbo Akademi, 1989.

Larsson, Maja. *Den moraliska kroppen: Tolkningar av kön och individualitet i 1800-talets populärmedicin*. Hedemora, Sweden: Gidlunds, 2002.

Latour, Bruno. *We Have Never Been Modern*. Cambridge, MA: Harvard University Press, 1993 [1991].

Le Cere del Museo dell'Istituto Fiorentino di Anatomia Patologica. Florence, Italy: Arnaud, [n.d.].

Leaney, Jennifer. "Ashes to Ashes: Cremation and the Celebration of Death in Nineteenth-Century Britain," in *Death, Ritual and Bereavement,* ed. Ralph Houlbrooke. London: Routledge, 1989.

Lennartsson, Rebecka. *Malaria Urbana—Om byråflickan Anna Johannesdotter och prostitutionen i Stockholm kring 1900.* Stockholm: Symposiun, 2001.

Lennmalm, Frithiof. *Svenska Läkaresällskapets historia 1808–1908.* Stockholm: Svenska läkaresällskapet, 1908.

Lepp, Hans. "Svenska Panoptikon," in *Sankt Eriks Årsbok 1978.* Stockholm, 1978.

Liedman, Sven-Eric. *Israel Hwasser.* Uppsala: Institutionen för idé- och lärdomshistoria, Uppsala universitet, 1971.

Lilja, Agneta. *Föreställningen om den ideala uppteckningen: En studie av idé och praktik vid traditionssamlande arkiv—ett exempel från Uppsala 1914–1945.* Uppsala: Dialekt- och fornminnesarkivet, Uppsala universitet, 1996.

Liljewall, Britt. *Självskrivna liv: Studier i äldre folkliga levnadsminnen.* Stockholm: Nordiska museets förlag, 2001.

Lindahl, Göran. *Grav och rum: Svenskt gravskick från medeltiden till 1800-talets slut.* Stockholm: Almqvist and Wiksell, 1969.

Ljungström, Olof. *Oscariansk antropologi: Etnografi, förhistoria och rasforskning under sent 1800-tal.* Hedemora, Sweden: Gidlunds, 2004.

Ljuva ögonblick—stunder av allvar, ed. Tommy Arvidsson and Birgit Brånvall. Stockholm: Nordiska museet, 1994.

MacDonald, Helen. *Human Remains: Episodes in Human Dissection.* Melbourne: Melbourne University Press, 2005.

Märker, Anna Katharina. "Model Experts: The Production and Uses of Anatomical Models at La Specola, Florence, and the Josephinum, Vienna, 1775–1814." Unpublished PhD dissertation, Ithaca, NY, Cornell University, 2005.

Maulitz, Russel C. *Morbid Appearances: The Anatomy of Pathology in the Early Nineteenth Century.* Cambridge: Cambridge University Press, 1987.

———. "The Pathological Tradition," in *Companion Encyclopedia of the History of Medicine,* ed. W. F. Bynum and Roy Porter. London: Routledge, 1993.

Medicine in the Twentieth Century, ed. Roger Cooter and John Pickstone. Amsterdam: Harwood Academic Publishers, 2000.

Meinwald, Dan. "Memento Mori: Death and Photography in Nineteenth Century America." http://vv.arts.ucla.edu/terminals/meinwald/meinwald1.html, accessed May 20, 2009.

Metcalf, Peter, and Richard Huntington. *Celebrations of Death: The Anthropology of Mortuary Ritual.* Cambridge: Cambridge University Press, 1991 [1979].

Mitford, Jessica. *The American Way of Death.* London: Hutchinson, 1963.

———. *The American Way of Death Revisited.* New York: Alfred A. Knopf, 1998.

Mjöberg, Lotte. *Femtio år i livets tjänst: Fonus i dag, i går, i morgon.* Stockholm: Informationsförlaget and Fonus, 1995.

Modärna tider: Vision och vardag i folkhemmet, ed. Jonas Frykman and Orvar Löfgren. Malmö, Sweden: Liber, 1985.

Modernity: An Introduction to Modern Societies, ed. S. Hall, D. Held, D. Hubert, and K. Thompson. Cambridge, MA: Blackwell, 1996.

Modernity and Technology, ed. T. J. Misa, P. Brey, and A. Feenberg. Cambridge, MA: MIT Press, 2003.

Monestier, Martin. *Peines de mort: Histoires et techniques des exécutions capitales des origines à nos jours.* Paris: Le cherche midi éditeur, 1994.

Motströms: Kritiken av det moderna, ed. Staffan Källström and Erland Sellberg. Stockholm: Carlssons, 1991.

Naar het lijk: Het Nederlandse doodsportret 1500-heden, ed. B. C. Sliggers. Haarlem, The Netherlands: Teylers Museum, 1998.

Nationalencyklopedin: Ett uppslagsverk på vetenskaplig grund utarbetat på initiativ av Statens kulturråd, ed. Kari Marklund et al. Höganäs, Sweden: Bra böcker, 1989.

Newall, Venetia. "Folklore and Cremation." *Folklore* 96, no. 2 (1985).

Nilsson, Gunnar. *Svenska Läkaresällskapets historia 1908–1938.* Stockholm: Svenska Generalstabens litografiska anstalts förlag, 1947.

Nilsson, Ulrika. "Att ta till kniven," in *Det givna och det föränderliga: En antologi om biologi, människobild och samhälle,* ed. Nils Uddenberg. Nora, Sweden: Nya Doxa, 2000.

———. *Det heta könet, Gynekologi i Sverige kring förra sekelskiftet.* Stockholm: Wahlström and Widstrand, 2005.

———. *Kampen om Kvinnan: Professionalisering och konstruktioner av kön i svensk gynekologi 1860–1925.* Uppsala: Institutionen för idé- och lärdomshistoria, Uppsala universitet, 2003.

———. "Kön, klass, och vetenskaplig auktoritet: Om kvinnliga läkarpionjärer," in *Vetenskapsbärarna: Naturvetenskapen i det svenska samhället 1880–1950,* ed. Sven Widmalm. Hedemora, Sweden: Gidlunds, 1999.

Nilsson, Ulrika, and Kristina Eriksson. "Kön och professionalisering: Om kvinnliga och manliga läkares strategier 1900 och 2000," in *Idéhistoriska perspektiv: Symposium i Göteborg, Arachne* 16, ed. Ingemar Nilsson. Göteborg: Institutionen för idéhistoria, Göteborgs universitet, 2000.

Nordenfelt, Lennart. *Causes of Death—A Philosophical Essay.* Stockholm: FRN, 1983.

Nordiska museet under 125 år, ed. Hans Medelius, Bengt Nyström, and Elisabet Stavenow-Hidemark. Stockholm: Nordiska museets förlag, 1998.

Nordström, Ingrid. "Begravningskalas," in *Dödens riter,* ed. Kristina Söderpalm. Stockholm: Carlssons, 1994.

Nouvelle Histoire de la Photographie, ed. Michel Frizot. Paris: Bordas, 1994.

Nylund Skog, Susanne. "Louise Hagberg som forskare och författare: En granskning av artikeln 'Julhalm och Juldockor' och des underlag." Unpublished thesis, Stockholm, Institutet för folklivsforskning, Stockholms universitet, 1993.

Odén, Birgitta, Bodil E.B. Persson, and Yvonne Maria Werner. *Den frivilliga döden: Samhällets hantering av självmord i historiskt perspektiv,* Stockholm: Cura and FRN, 1998.

Ohlander, Ann-Sofie. "'Den smärtsamma oro, vilken bragt honom ända till ledsnad vid livet': Synen på självmord i Sverige från medeltid till 1900-tal," in *Kärlek, död och frihet: Historiska uppsatser om människovärde och livsvillkor i Sverige.* Stockholm: Norstedts, 1986.

Olsson, Ingrid. *Att leva som lytt: Handikappades levnadsvillkor i 1800-talets Linköping.* Linköping, Sweden: Institutionen för Tema, Linköpings universitet, 1999.

Parsons, Brian. *Committed to the Flame: The Development of Cremation in Nineteenth-Century England*. Reading: Spire Books, 2005.

Persson, Bodil. *När kvinnorna kom in i männens värld: Framväxten av ett kvinnligt tekniskt yrke—laboratorieassistent under perioden 1880–1941*. Malmö, Sweden: Vårdförbundet SHSTF, 1994.

Picturing Knowledge: Historical and Philosophical Problems Concerning the Use of Art in Science, ed. Brian S. Baigrie. Toronto: University of Toronto Press, 1996.

Pleijel, Hilding. *Jordfästning i stillhet: Från samhällsstraff till privat-ceremoni: En samhällshistorisk studie*. Lund: Arken, 1983.

Porter, Roy. *Bodies Politic: Disease, Death, and Doctors in Britain 1650–1900*. Ithaca, NY: Cornell University Press, 2001.

Pressac, Jean-Claude. *Krematorierne i Auschwitz: Massedrapets maskineri*. Oslo: Aventura, 1994.

Prothero, Stephen. *Purified by Fire: A History of Cremation in America*. Berkeley: University of California Press, 2001.

The Quick and the Dead: Artists and Anatomy, ed. Deanna Petheridge and Ludmilla Jordanova. London: National Touring Exhibitions, 1997.

Quigley, Christine. *The Corpse: A History*. Jefferson, NC: McFarland, 1996.

Qvarsell, Roger. "Inledning," in *I framtidens tjänst: Ur folkhemmets idéhistoria*, ed. Roger Qvarsell. Stockholm: Gidlunds, 1986.

———. *Utan vett och vilja: Om synen på brottslighet och sinnesjukdom*. Stockholm: Carlssons, 1993.

———. *Vårdens idéhistoria*. Stockholm: Carlssons, 1991.

Rehnberg, Mats. *Ljusen på gravarna och andra ljusseder: Nya traditioner under 1900-talet*. Stockholm: Nordiska museet, 1965.

Reklam och hälsa: Levnadsideal, skönhet och hälsa i den svenska reklamens historia, ed. Roger Qvarsell and Ulrika Torell. Stockholm: Carlssons, 2005.

Richardson, Ruth. *Death, Dissection, and the Destitute*. London: Routledge and Kegan Paul, 1987.

Ricoeur, Paul. *Från text till handling: En antologi om hermeneutik*, ed. Peter Kemp and Bengt Kristensson. Stockholm: Symposion, 1988 [1986].

———. "Le temps raconté." *Revue de Métaphysique et de Morale* 4 (1984).

Ristilammi, Per-Markku. "The Bodily Eye: Reflections on the Era of the Stereoscope," in *Amalgamations: Fusing Technology and Culture*, ed. Susanne Lundin and Lynn Åkesson. Lund: Nordic Acadmic Press, 1999.

———. "Optiska illusioner—fetischism mellan modernitet och primitivism." *Kulturella perspektiv* 3 (1995).

Ritvo, Harriet. *The Platypus and the Mermaid, and Other Figments of the Classifying Imagination*. Cambridge, MA: Harvard University Press, 1997.

Roberts, K. B., and J.D.W. Tomlinson. *The Fabric of the Body: European Traditions of Anatomical Illustration*. Oxford: Clarendon, 1992.

Roberts, Russell. "Taxonomi: Om fotografins och klassificeringens historia," in *I skuggan av ljuset: Fotografi och systematik i konst, vetenskap och vardagsliv*. Stockholm: Moderna museet, 1998.

Rocca, Julius. *Forging a Medical University: The Establishment of Sweden's Karolinska Institutet*. Stockholm: Karolinska Institutet University Press, 2006.

Rosen, Fred. *Cremation in America*. Amherst, MA: Prometheus Books, 2004.

Ruby, Jay. *Secure the Shadow: Death and Photography in America.* Cambridge, MA: MIT Press, 1995.

Rundquist, Angela. *Blått blod och liljevita händer: En etnologisk studie av aristokratiska kvinnor 1850–1900.* Stockholm: Carlssons, 1989.

———. "Hovfruntimret—ett nobelt ykeskollektiv 1850–1900." *Livrustkammaren* 17, nos. 5–6 (1986).

Runeby, Nils. *Teknikerna, vetenskapen, och kulturen: Ingenjörsundervisning och ingenjörsorganisationer i 1870-talets Sverige.* Uppsala: Institutionen för idé- och lärdomshistoria, Uppsala universitet, 1976.

Russett, Cynthia Eagle. *Sexual Science: The Victorian Construction of Womanhood.* Cambridge, MA: Harvard University Press, 1989.

Saban, Roger, and Sylvie Hughes. "Les Musée d'anatomie de l'institut d'anatomie." *Histoire des Science Médicales* 33, no. 2 (1999).

"Sam. Lindskog, Kgl. Hoffotograf, Örebro," in *Från bergslag och bondebygd 1983,* ed. Egon Thun. Örebro, Sweden: Örebro läns hembygdsförbund and Stiftelsen Örebro läns museum, 1983.

Sandberg, Mark B. *Living Pictures, Missing Persons: Mannequins, Museums and Modernity.* Princeton: Princeton University Press, 2003.

Sappol, Michael. *A Traffic of Dead Bodies: Anatomy and Embodied Social Identity in Nineteenth-Century America.* Princeton: Princeton University Press, 2002.

Sawday, Jonathan. *The Body Emblazoned: Dissection and the Human Body in Renaissance Culture.* London: Routledge, 1995.

Schiebinger, Londa. *Nature's Body: Gender in the Making of Modern Science.* Boston: Beacon, 1993.

Schilling, Chris. *The Body and Social Theory.* London: Sage, 1993.

Schlosser, Julius von. "Geschichte der Porträtbildnerei in Wachs: Ein Versuch," in *Jahrbuch der Kunsthistorische Sammlungen d. allerh. Kaiserhauses* 29, no. 3. Vienna, 1911.

Schwartz, Vanessa R. *Spectacular Realities: Early Mass Culture in Fin-de-Siècle Paris.* Berkeley: University of California Press, 1998.

Sedgwick, Eve Kosofsky. *Between Men: English Literature and Male Homosocial Desire.* New York: University of Columbia Press, 1985.

"Send us a Lady Physician": Women Doctors in America, 1835–1920, ed. Ruth J. Abram. New York: W. W. Norton, 1985.

Showalter, Elaine. *Sexual Anarchy: Gender and Culture at the Fin-de-Siècle.* London: Bloomsbury, 1991.

Sidén, Karin. *Den ideala barndomen: Studier i det stormaktstida barnporträttets ikonografi och funktion.* Stockholm: Raster, 2001.

———. "Porträtt av döda," in *Ansikte mot ansikte: Porträtt från fem sekel,* ed. Görel Cavalli-Björkman. Stockholm Nationalmuseum/Atlantis, 2001.

Skarin Frykman, Birgitta. "Det skulle visas utåt att man hade lik i huset . . . ," in *Dödens riter,* ed. Kristina Söderpalm. Stockholm: Carlsson, 1994.

Snickare, Mårten. *Enväldets riter: Kungliga fester och ceremonier i gestaltning av Nicodemus Tessin den yngre.* Stockholm: Raster, 1999.

Snickars, Pelle. *Svensk film och tidig visuell masskultur 1900.* Stockholm: Aura förlag, 2001.

Söderberg, Rolf. *Stockholmsgryning: En fotografisk vandring på Karl XV:s tid.* Stockholm: Liber, 1986.

Söderberg, Rolf, and Pär Rittsel. *Den svenska fotografins historia.* Stockholm: Bonnier-Fakta, 1983.

Söderlind, Solfrid. *Porträttbruk i Sverige 1840–1865.* Stockholm: Carlssons, 1994.

———. "Privat objekt och offentligt medium: Kungligt porträttbruk i Sverige—tidiga fotografiska bilder," in *Fotobilden: Historien i nuet—nuet i historien,* ed. Lena Johannesson, Angelika Sjölander-Hovorka, and Solfrid Söderlind. Linköping, Sweden: Institutionen för Tema, Linköpings universitet, 1989.

Sommestad, Lena. *Från mejerska till mejerist: En studie av mejeriyrkets maskuliniserings-process.* Lund: Arkiv, 1992.

Sörlin, Sverker. "Utopin i verkligheten: Ludvig Nordström och det moderna Sverige," in *I framtidens tjänst: ur folkhemmets idéhistoria,* ed. Roger Qvarsell. Stockholm: Gidlunds, 1986.

Stafford, Barbara Maria. *Artful Science: Enlightenment Entertainment and the Eclipse of Visual Education.* Cambridge, MA: MIT Press, 1994.

———. *Body Criticism: Imaging the Unseen in Enlightenment Art and Medicine.* Cambridge, MA: MIT Press, 1997 [1991].

Stannard, David E. *The Puritan Way of Death: A Study in Religion, Culture, and Social Change.* Oxford: Oxford University Press, 1977.

Star, Susan Leigh, and James R. Griesemer. "Insitutional Ecology, 'Translations' and Boundary Objects: Amateurs and Professionals in Berkeley's Museum of Verte-brate Zoology, 1907–1939." *Social Studies of Science* 19 (1989).

Stepan, Nancy. *The Idea of Race in Science: Great Britain 1800–1960.* London: Macmillan, 1982.

Tellgren, Anna. *Tio fotografer: Självsyn och bildsyn: Svensk fotografi under 1950-talet i ett internationellt perspektiv.* Stockholm: Informationsförlaget, 1997.

Thomasson, Peter. "Eldbegängelsens teknikhistoria." Unpublished undergraduate thesis, Stockholm, Avdelningen för teknikhistoria, KTH, 1987.

Thomson, Rosemarie Garland. *Extraordinary Bodies: Figuring Physical Disability in Amer-ican Culture and Literature.* New York: Columbia University Press, 1997.

Thor, Clas. *Ljusets hemligheter: Kvinnligt fotografi 1861–1986.* Örebro, Sweden: Mor-gonstjärnan, 1986.

Thörn, Håkan. *Modernitet, sociologi och sociala rörelser.* Göteborg: Sociologiska institu-tionen, Göteborgs universitet, 1997.

———. *Rörelser i det moderna: Politik, modernitet och kollektiv identitet i Europa 1789–1989.* Stockholm: Tiden/Athena, 1997.

Tjerneld, Staffan. *Stockholmsliv: Hur vi bott, arbetat och roat oss under 100 år: Med bidrag av stockholmsforskare, författare och journalister I–II.* Stockholm: Norstedts, 1949–50.

Turner, Bryan S. *Theories of Modernity and Postmodernity.* London: Sage, 1990.

Turner, Victor. *The Anthropology of Performance.* New York: PAJ, 1986.

———. *Dramas, Fields, and Metaphors: Symbolic Action in Human Society.* Ithaca, NY: Cor-nell University Press, 1974.

Verdier, Yvonne. *Façons de dire, façons de faire: La laveuse, la couturière, la cuisinière.* Paris: Gallimard, 1979.

———. *Tvätterskan, kokerskan, sömmerskan: Livet i en fransk by genom tre kvinnoyrken.* Stockholm: Atlantis, 1981.

Vetenskapsbärarna: Naturvetenskapen i det svenska samhället 1880–1950, ed. Sven Widmalm. Hedemora, Sweden: Gidlunds, 1999.

Vovelle, Michel. *La mort et l'Occident de 1300 à nos jours.* Paris: Gallimard, 1983.

———. *Mourir autrefois: Attitudes collectives devant la mort aux XVIIe et XVIIIe siècles.* Paris: Gallimard, 1974.

Walter, Tony. *The Revival of Death.* London: Routledge, 1994.

Warner, John Harley. *Against the Spirit of System: The French Impulse in Nineteenth-Century American Medicine.* Baltimore: Johns Hopkins University Press, 1998.

Warner, John Harley and James M. Edmonson. *Dissection: Photographs of a Rite of Passage in American Medicine, 1880–1930.* New York: Blast Books, 2009.

Warner, John Harley, and Lawrence J. Rizzolo. "Anatomical Instruction and Training for Professionalism from the 19th to the 21st Centuries." *Clinical Anatomy* 19 (2006).

Waugh, Evelyn. *The Loved One: An Anglo-American Tragedy.* London: Penguin, 1951 [1948].

Weber, Max. *The Protestant Ethic and the Spirit of Capitalism.* New York: Scribner's, 1958 [1905].

Weimarck, Torsten. *Akademi och anatomi: Några aspekter på människokroppens historia i nya tidens konstnärsutbildning med tonvikt på anatomiundervisning vid konstakademierna i Stockholm och Köpenhamn fram till 1800-talets början.* Stockholm: Symposion, 1996.

———. *Den normala kroppen: Några förvandlingar i bildkonsten av ett anatomiskt motiv.* Stockholm: Symposion, 1989.

White, Hayden. *Metahistory: The Historical Imagination in Nineteenth Century Europe.* Baltimore: Johns Hopkins University Press, 1978.

———. *Tropics of Discourse: Essays in Cultural Criticism.* Baltimore: Johns Hopkins University Press, 1978.

Wikander, Ulla. *Delat arbete, delad makt; om kvinnans underordning i och genom arbetet: En historisk essä.* Uppsala: Institutionen för ekonomisk historia, Uppsala universitet, 1991.

Wikman, K. Robert V. "Louise Hagberg †," in *Fataburen: Nordiska museets och Skansens årsbok.* Stockholm, 1945.

Wolf-Knuts, Ulrika. "Liktvättning—ett kvinnoarbete," in *Budkavlen.* Åbo, Finland: Åbo Akademi, 1983.

Young, Katharine. *Presence in the Flesh: The Body in Medicine.* Cambridge, MA: Harvard University Press, 1997.

Index

Page numbers in italics refer to figures.